PUBLIC HEALTH IN THE 21ST CENTURY

WEIGHT GAIN

WOMEN'S ATTITUDES, HEALTH IMPLICATIONS AND PSYCHOLOGICAL CHALLENGES

PUBLIC HEALTH IN THE 21ST CENTURY

Additional books in this series can be found on Nova's website under the Series tab.

Additional e-books in this series can be found on Nova's website under the e-book tab.

PUBLIC HEALTH IN THE 21ST CENTURY

WEIGHT GAIN

WOMEN'S ATTITUDES, HEALTH IMPLICATIONS AND PSYCHOLOGICAL CHALLENGES

ALESSIO PIROTTE
AND
TRISTAN LIBERT
EDITORS

NOVINKA

New York

For permission to use material from this book please contact us:
Telephone 631-231-7269; Fax 631-231-8175
Web Site: http://www.novapublishers.com

NOTICE TO THE READER

Library of Congress Cataloging-in-Publication Data

ISBN: 978-1-62618-800-6

Published by Nova Science Publishers, Inc. † New York

CONTENTS

PREFACE

In this book, the authors discuss women's attitudes, the health implications and psychological challenges of weight gain. Topics include whether exercise training can reduce the prevalence of obesity with a high-fat diet; women's body image and weight gain in pregnancy; maternal weight gain and perinatal outcomes; and women's perceptions of postpartum weight retention and their body image in relation to breastfeeding outcomes in Japan.

Chapter 1 – *Introduction:* Pregnancy is a time of tremendous physiological change wherein weight gain is of biologic importance. For most women this is an important and inevitable factor for healthy gestation. This increase in weight occurs over a short period of time, which may be perceived by pregnant women with either a positive or negative attitude.

Objective: The goal for this chapter is to provide an assessment of body image, weight gain and associated attitudes towards weight gain during pregnancy using a prospective study that follows pregnant woman over the course of their pregnancy. Specifically, to i) examine how the different factors, including women's attitudes, may affect weight gain and self-esteem (e.g. body image) in relation to maternal characteristics: parity, pre-pregnancy BMI (normal weight, overweight, obese) and gestational weight gain (adequate versus excessive); ii) investigate temporal patterns in gestational weight gain and its associated eating-related attitudes across 3 times points in pregnancy; and iii) assess adequacy of total gestational weight gain (GWG) between the pre-pregnancy BMI categories in relation the updated 2009 Institute of Medicine (IOM) guidelines.

Results: As measured by the Pregnancy Experience Scale (PES), both parity groups saw an increase in frequency of uplifts over the course of pregnancy but there were no significant differences between nulli- and primi/multiparous women. Nulliparous women had a lower PES composite ratio score (intensity of hassles/intensity of uplifts) vs. multiparous (0.68 ± 0.013 vs. 0.78 ± 0.015, $p=0.011$). Pregnancy and Weight Gain Attitude Scale (PWGAS) scores increased over time in both parity groups with no difference in mean score. A greater number of nulliparous women reported not being embarrassed by the weight they had gained, but after adjustment for covariates this became non-significant ($p=0.065$). According to PES scores, women in all BMI categories reported an increasing number of uplifts over time with no between group differences. Similarly there were no differences across the BMI groups in their PWGAS score over the course of pregnancy. Those women who met IOM guidelines for GWG had significantly more positive weight gain attitudes ($p=0.012$). Overweight and obese women reported a stronger diet history than normal weight women (as measured frequency of past dieting, attempts to lose 10 kg or more etc.) Overweight women had significantly higher GWG vs. obese women over pregnancy ($p<0.016$). Both overweight and obese women exceeded the recommended rate of weight gain in the 2nd and 3rd trimester.

Conclusions: Overall, examining body image and how it relates to eating behaviour and weight gain in pregnancy is a clinically relevant discussion topic and important area of research given healthy dietary and weight management behaviours are known to positively influence mom and baby.

Chapter 2 – Weight gain management before and during pregnancy may be a key factor influencing the health of women during pregnancy and the development of the fetus. Adequate gestational weight gain contributes to better pregnancy outcomes in both mothers and infants, in short- and long-term. The Institute of Medicine (IOM) released gestational weight guidelines for optimal pregnancy outcomes. The guideline will be used in clinical practices for effective weight management aiming at improving fetal and maternal outcomes.

Evidences from human and animal studies of pre-pregnancy body mass index and gestational weight gain showed that altering the environment of utero could lead to lifelong health consequences, such as high adiposity, sarcopenia, insulin resistance, glucose intolerance, and high blood pressure. Population-based prospective cohort studies starting from different geographical regions in the pre-conceptional period or in early fetal life, in which the offspring is followed from early fetal life until young adulthood. All women of reproductive age are encouraged to follow the IOM recommendations and maintain a well-balanced diet. To improve birth outcomes, it is critical for women to modify their health behaviors for a better nutritional status before, during, and after conception.

Chapter 3 – Weight retention in the postpartum period is a concern for many women following the increase in weight during pregnancy and they often struggle to return to pre-pregnancy levels. Postpartum weight retention may lead to obesity that is then associated with increased rates of several chronic diseases, including type 2 diabetes and cardiovascular disease. Prolonged breastfeeding is believed to help with weight loss during the postpartum period. Breastfeeding and in particular, 'exclusive breastfeeding' for the first six month of life, provides a wide range of health benefits for infants but also to mothers. Most pediatric organizations recommend exclusive breastfeeding for six months and then continuing for as long as the mother desires.

In Japan, women's body image has a strong influence on control of their weight due to the prevailing cultural norm that 'being slim is beautiful'. This is an important factor when considering postpartum weight retention together with breastfeeding practices. Japan has the least number of women who are overweight among all of the developed countries. But despite this many Japanese women perceive themselves to be overweight, both before and after pregnancy. While they of necessity increase their weight during pregnancy, many undertake activities to regain pre-pregnancy body shape soon after birth due to their desire to regain their ideal body image of being slim. A study of Japanese postpartum women residing in Himeji-city, (n = 1,612) showed that more than 42% of women believed that they had not yet returned to their weight at 18 months postpartum, even though 18% were actually in the 'underweight range (Body Mass Index ≤ 18.5)'. The women who had returned to their pre-pregnancy weight stated that their weight loss usually occurred within six months after birth (59.6%), during the time when most were breastfeeding. In the study, the postpartum women were asked about their level of concern about body appearance using the Attention to Body Shape Scale (ABS). The average score of the ABS was 24.2 (Standard Deviation [SD] = 4.2) suggesting that postpartum women in Japan were highly conscious about their body shape. Women's body image is related to infant feeding practices as breastfeeding is associated with weight loss, but also breastfeeding may be associated with breast shape changes and hence changes in body image. In this chapter, the authors describe and discuss women's perceptions of postpartum weight retention and their body image in relation to breastfeeding outcomes, particularly focusing on a trend in Japan.

Chapter 4 – High-fat diet induces obesity. It is considered as the second most lethal habit after smoking. The purpose of this study was to examine the effect of exercise training on the control of weight gain in rats receiving fat diet.

The study was carried out with three groups of rats (n=12); the standard diet sedentary group (SS) (control group), standard diet with exercise (SE) and high fat diet with exercise (FE). Animals in high fat diet group were fed a diet containing 10% olive oil (weight/weight). Trained rats swam 1 hour/day 5 times weekly for 4 weeks.

Significant reductions in weight gain and in food intake were observed with training ($p<0.001$). Body weight was maintained in trained rats receiving fat diet. Fat diet significantly increased both insulin concentrations ($p<0.05$), glycaemia ($p<0.001$) and muscle glycogen ($p<0.001$).

This research demonstrated the efficient effect of exercise training on preventing overweight in rats fed fat diet. The authors' results showed, as well, the positive effect of physical exercise on reducing both food intake and weight gain.

In: Weight Gain
Editors: A. Pirotte and T. Libert
ISBN: 978-1-62618-800-6

Chapter 1

WEIGHT GAIN, BODY IMAGE AND ATTITUDES OVER THE COURSE OF PREGNANCY

Kristi B. Adamo[1,2,3,*]***, Sonia Jean-Philippe***[1]***, Shanna Wilson***[1]***, Zachary M. Ferraro***[1]***, Irene Strychar***[4]***, Kara Nerenberg***[5] ***and Gary Goldfield***[1,2,3]

[1]Children's Hospital of Eastern Ontario Research Institute, Healthy Active Living and Obesity Research Group, Ottawa, Canada
[2]University of Ottawa, Faculty of Medicine, Pediatrics, Canada
[3]University of Ottawa, Faculty of Health Sciences, School of Human Kinetics, Ottawa, Canada
[4]Université de Montréal, Centre de recherche du Centre Hospitalier de l'Université de Montréal, Hôpital Notre-Dame du CHUM, Montréal, Canada
[5]University of Ottawa, Division of General Internal Medicine, Ottawa, Canada

ABSTRACT

Introduction: Pregnancy is a time of tremendous physiological change wherein weight gain is of biologic importance. For most women

---

* Corresponding author: E-mail: kadamo@cheo.on.ca.

this is an important and inevitable factor for healthy gestation. This increase in weight occurs over a short period of time, which may be perceived by pregnant women with either a positive or negative attitude.

Objective: The goal for this chapter is to provide an assessment of body image, weight gain and associated attitudes towards weight gain during pregnancy using a prospective study that follows pregnant woman over the course of their pregnancy. Specifically, to i) examine how the different factors, including women's attitudes, may affect weight gain and self-esteem (e.g. body image) in relation to maternal characteristics: parity, pre-pregnancy BMI (normal weight, overweight, obese) and gestational weight gain (adequate versus excessive); ii) investigate temporal patterns in gestational weight gain and its associated eating-related attitudes across 3 times points in pregnancy; and iii) assess adequacy of total gestational weight gain (GWG) between the pre-pregnancy BMI categories in relation the updated 2009 Institute of Medicine (IOM) guidelines.

Results: As measured by the Pregnancy Experience Scale (PES), both parity groups saw an increase in frequency of uplifts over the course of pregnancy but there were no significant differences between nulli- and primi/multiparous women. Nulliparous women had a lower PES composite ratio score (intensity of hassles/intensity of uplifts) vs. multiparous (0.68 ± 0.013 vs. 0.78 ± 0.015, $p=0.011$). Pregnancy and Weight Gain Attitude Scale (PWGAS) scores increased over time in both parity groups with no difference in mean score. A greater number of nulliparous women reported not being embarrassed by the weight they had gained, but after adjustment for covariates this became non-significant ($p=0.065$). According to PES scores, women in all BMI categories reported an increasing number of uplifts over time with no between group differences. Similarly there were no differences across the BMI groups in their PWGAS score over the course of pregnancy. Those women who met IOM guidelines for GWG had significantly more positive weight gain attitudes ($p=0.012$). Overweight and obese women reported a stronger diet history than normal weight women (as measured frequency of past dieting, attempts to lose 10 kg or more etc.) Overweight women had significantly higher GWG vs. obese women over pregnancy ($p<0.016$). Both overweight and obese women exceeded the recommended rate of weight gain in the 2nd and 3rd trimester.

Conclusions: Overall, examining body image and how it relates to eating behaviour and weight gain in pregnancy is a clinically relevant discussion topic and important area of research given healthy dietary and weight management behaviours are known to positively influence mom and baby.

DEFINITIONS

Primigravida = A woman pregnant for the first time.
Nulliparous= A woman in her first pregnancy and who has not yet given birth is a nullipara or nullip. After she gives birth she becomes primiparous.

Primiparous = A woman who has given birth once before is primiparous, and would be referred to as a primipara or primip.

Multiparous = A woman who has given birth two or more times is multiparous and is called a multip.

INTRODUCTION

Weight gain is natural, important part of pregnancy. Over a short period of time, women's bodies undergo several physical and biological changes. Unfortunately for many women, these changes can results in potentially uncomfortable side effects (e.g., nausea, swelling, joint pain etc.). It has been suggested that a woman's attitude, including perception of body image, may have an impact on the amount of weight she gains during pregnancy [1-3]. According to Cash [4], body image is defined as a "multifaceted psychological experience of embodiment, especially but not exclusively one's physical appearance; it encompasses one's body-related self-perceptions and self-attitudes, including thoughts, beliefs, feelings and behaviours". An understanding of body satisfaction is important given that discontentment with one's body may lead to disordered eating behaviours such as fasting, binging with or without purging or dieting while pregnant [5]. These unhealthy eating behaviours are linked to inadequate weight gain, premature delivery, low birth weight, and delayed child development [5-8]. Meanwhile, qualitative research has noted that women may see the changes associated with pregnancy as "transient" and "unique to the childbearing experience" allowing them to accept these changes without distress [9]. For example, a woman may feel less pressure to internalize weight biases during this period as she sees herself as playing an important reproductive role [10, 11]. Attitudes related to food and dieting -pre-pregnancy may also result from a woman's desire to achieve her ideal perceived body type which may carry over into pregnancy. Indeed, habitual dieters or restrictors within normal, overweight and obese categories may gain above the recommended guidelines while underweight women may gain below recommendations [12]. While there is evidence demonstrating that habitual dieters may feel less accountable for their weight while pregnant [13, 14], others have argued that the widespread aversion to being "fat" among the female population may prejudice women against gaining weight during their pregnancy [2]. Since body image and fear of weight gain may contribute to pregnancy eating and dieting behaviours, it is fundamental to address this topic as appropriate gestational weight gain is paramount for maternal and fetal health in the short and long term [15].

Why Is Gestational Weight Gain an Important Concern?

Insufficient or excessive weight gain can compromise the health of both mother and baby. However, in today's obesogenic environment, excessive weight gain is much more common. In fact, excessive weight gain is frequent in women of all BMI categories. This presents a challenge as maternal pre-pregnancy BMI and gestational weight gain (GWG) have been recognized as vital contributing factors to child obesity. Both are positively associated with infant birth weight [16-20], as well as child and adult BMI, and more recently evidence suggesting a relationship between gestational weight gain and downstream overweight/obesity in children has been published [21-23]. Although excess GWG is contraindicated in all women, the risks are amplified in overweight and obese women. Between 1993 and 2003, pre-pregnancy obesity increased by 69% in the US from 13% to 22% [24] and, over a similar time frame the proportion of women in the obese categories increased from 3% to 10% in the Canadian population [25]. In North America, approximately 54.5% of women of childbearing age (20-39 years) are overweight, 29% are classified as obese and 6% are considered morbidly obese [26]. Recommended total gestational weight gain guidelines from the Institutes of Medicine are shown in Table 1 [27]. From observational studies conducted in the United-States, roughly 30-40% of women gained weight within the recommended ranges, 20% gained less, and 40-50% gained more than what is recommended [28]. In a Canadian regional analysis (i.e., the Ottawa and Kingston (OaK) birth cohort), 27, 47, 78 and 72% of underweight, normal weight, overweight and obese women gained in excess of the 2009 IOM weight gain recommendations, while 21, 17, 4 and 11%, respectively, gained below the guidelines [29].

Table 1. Recommended rate of weight gain and total GWG for pregnancy, stratified by pre-pregnancy BMI category, according to the 2009 IOM recommendations [27]

Pre-pregnancy BMI category	IOM guideline	
	Mean rate of weight gain in the 2nd and 3rd trimester (kg/wk) [a]	Total weight gain (kg)
Normal weight: BMI = 18.5 - 24.9	0.4	11.5 – 16.0
Overweight: BMI = 25.0 - 29.9	0.3	7.0 - 11.5
Obese: BMI ≥ 30	0.2	5.0 – 9.0

Legend: BMI, Body Mass Index; IOM, Institute of Medicine.
[a] In the first trimester, there is an assumed range of weight gain of 0.5 – 2 kg.

Along with the increased obesity prevalence in women of child bearing age, a higher pre-pregnancy BMI and higher GWG are associated with many health risks during pregnancy, including greater incidence of developing preeclampsia and gestational diabetes mellitus (GDM) [19, 30-35].

The Assessment of Body Image throughout the Decades

Over the course of the last 30 years, body image has been assessed using both qualitative and quantitative approaches. Various questionnaires have been created and validated to quantitatively assess body image, weight gain attitudes and eating behaviours. Body image questionnaires that have been used in pregnancy research are outlined in Table 2.

The '70s and '80s

As early as 1977, it was reported that some women may develop a particularly distorted body image during pregnancy [48]. This was later supported by a retrospective study evaluating women before, during and after pregnancy [49].

Table 2. Qualitative and quantitative questionnaires for assessing body image, weight gain attitudes and eating behaviours during pregnancy

Authors	Questionnaire	Description
Cooper et al., 1987	Eating Disorder Examination-Questionnaire (EDE-Q) [36]	Measures key behavioral and attitudinal features including overeating; dieting; self-induced vomiting; laxative misuse; and concerns about eating, shape, and weight.
Thompson, 1996	Body Image Satisfaction (BIS) [37]	Score derived from the Figure Rating Scale, which presents images of nine figures ranging from very thin to very heavy. Discrepancy between the figure selected as ideal and current body size are utilized as the BIS score.
Palmer et al., 1985	Pregnancy and Weight Gain Attitude Scale (PWGAS) [2]	Measures attitude towards weight gain during pregnancy.
DiPietro et al., 2004	Pregnancy Experience Scale (PES) [38]	Measures maternal appraisal of exposure to daily, ongoing hassles and uplifts which are specific to pregnancy (e.g., 'Discussing baby names with your spouse,' 'Making nursery arrangements,' 'Physical symptoms'). The PES structure was modeled on the non-pregnancy Hassles and Uplifts Scale [39].
Cooper et al., 1987	Body Shape Questionnaire (BSQ) – 34 items [40]	Measures concern with body shape over the last four weeks in areas such as clothing, socializing, and eating (e.g., Have you avoided situations where people could see your body? Has seeing your reflection made you feel bad about your shape?). Responses are marked on a 6-point scale from "Never experiencing" to "Always experiencing." Higher scores indicate more negative body shape concerns.
Secord and Jourard, 1953	Body Cathexis Scale [41]	Original BCS contains 46 items with a 5-point response scale to measure the function of the body parts and the patient's satisfaction with this function.
Mirucka, 2005	Body Image Questionnaire [42] assesses body image along four dimensions	Acceptance of one's body, disclosure of femininity, experience of intimate relations with persons of the opposite sex, attitude towards eating and body weight.

Authors	**Questionnaire**	**Description**
Garner and Garfinkel, 1979	Eating Attitudes Test (EAT) [43]	26-item self-report measure used to identify eating disturbances in both clinical and nonclinical populations, it assesses eating disorder risk. 3 subscales: dieting, bulimia and food preoccupation, oral control.
Pingitore et al., 1997	Body Shape Satisfaction Scale [44]	10 items assessing satisfaction with different body parts with five Likert response categories ranging from very dissatisfied to very satisfied.
Williamson et al., 2000	Body Image Assessment for Obesity Tool (BIA-O) [45]	Measures ideal and current body sizes Using silhouettes of men and women ranging from very thin to very obese.
Van Strien et al., 1986	Dutch Eating Behaviour Questionnaire (DEBQ) [46]	Consists of three different scales to measure eating behaviour including the following: emotional, external and restrained eating. All of the items are rated on a five-point Likert scale with a rating of one ('never') to five ('very often). Of note: the emotional eating scale can be broken down into two different subscales
Stunkard and Messick, 1985	Three Factor Eating Questionnaire (TFEQ) [47]	Consists of 51 questions and measures three dimensions of human eating behavior: cognitive restraint of eating, disinhibition and hunger. Each item scores either 0 or 1 point. The minimum score for factors I-II-III is therefore 0-0-0, the possible maximum score 21-16-14.

Sixty-three women were assessed using a modified version of the *Attitude to Body Image Scale*, which provides a list of body parts for which women indicate their attitude towards each using a Likert-scale. The participants felt significantly more negative about their bodies during the last three months of pregnancy than they did before the onset of their pregnancy and post-partum [49]. The multiparas had a more positive attitude toward their body image than did the primiparas. The authors suggested that multiparous women's priorities may shift to increased concerns over having sufficient energy to meet the demands of daily responsibilities of tending to the family rather than focusing on the changes and physical appearance of her body [49]. In the 80s, Palmer and colleagues developed the *Pregnancy and Weight Gain Attitude Scale,* to determine if there was a potential association between attitudes and actual weight gain during pregnancy [2]. They found a significant association between the attitude score and actual weight gain such that attitudes favouring slimness may be associated with smaller weight gain during pregnancy [2]. However, in the 70's and 80's, research examining attitudes around pregnancy related weight gain, body image and associated eating behaviours became an emerging new field of study.

The 90s

This decade saw a burgeoning of research in this area and early on, Fairburn and Welch interviewed first time mothers within days of giving birth and categorized them by their pre-pregnancy dieting history (dieter vs. non-dieter) [1]. Most women participating in this qualitative study reported eating more often during than prior to pregnancy. The authors suggested three reasons for these changes: i) overeating may relieve nausea; ii) eating 'little and often' minimised the experience of fullness in the third trimester; and iii) the belief that increased frequency of eating may be beneficial to the health of the baby. Overall, nearly half the women expressed no concern about the increase in their weight and 30% felt a lessening in their usual weight concerns. Three quarters of those who were afraid of gaining an excessive amount of weight were from the pre-pregnancy dieting group. The dieting group also reacted more negatively than the non-dieting group to the changes in their shape, with few responding positively. The findings of this study indicated that women who were previously concerned about their shape, weight, or eating, as judged by their diet history, differ in their psychological response by exhibiting greater body image concern to pregnancy from those who did not have such eating-related concerns. Shortly after, Fairburn and colleagues completed a prospective study of 100 primigravid women examining the pregnancy related changes in eating behaviour [14]. They assessed clinical features of eating disorders using the *Eating Disorder Examination* (EDE) questionnaire and found a significant change in the degree of concern about body shape across the trimesters. Notably, this work detected a decline in the level of concern about weight in the early stages of pregnancy, followed by an increase in later gestation. Fairburn's group had previously hypothesized that weight concerns may decrease in early pregnancy when women feel less accountable for their weight [1] while increased concern towards the end of the pregnancy may be related to the fear of not returning to their pre-pregnancy weight. However, this latter study lacked a comparison group such as non-pregnant or multiparous women, which prevents clear conclusions from being made.

Using a retrospective design, Abraham and colleagues assessed 100 primigravid women using an eating behaviour questionnaire and showed that 73% of women who had used some 'healthful' (sensible exercise routines, avoiding eating between meals, avoiding certain foods) or 'detrimental' weight control measures (dieting, self-induced vomiting, laxatives, starvation) before pregnancy continued to use these during pregnancy [50]. This team explored the value of weighing women throughout pregnancy and almost half (n=46) of the participants felt that being weighed resulted in adopting healthier eating patterns [50]. In contrast to the previous studies, Davies and Wardle compared 76 pregnant women to a control non-pregnant group (n=97) and found that pregnant women were less dissatisfied with their bodies than non-pregnant women, however they did not differ in their choices of body image ideals. These results indicate that while there may be an easing of current body image fears during pregnancy and a transition to a state of greater acceptance, the underlying cognition of their preferred or ideal body image remains strong [51].

Further work that compared primigravid to non-pregnant nulliparous women (n=100) looked at the relationship between disordered eating and body image using several assessment tools including the *Dutch Eating Behaviour Questionnaire* (DEBQ), *Eating Self-Efficacy Scale* (ESES), *Three Factor Eating Questionnaire* (TFEQ) and the *Body Shape Questionnaire* (BSQ). This work supported the notion that pregnant women at 24-28 weeks report greater satisfaction with their body shape than non-pregnant women [13] and data from a subgroup of restrained eaters indicated that pregnant restrained eaters reported significantly less restraint in their eating than the non-pregnant restrained eaters. These data point toward a relaxation of restrictive eating behaviours during pregnancy for women who would generally try to control their intake. It must be noted that these results contrast with earlier work by Slade PD in 1977 and Strang and Sullivan in 1985 [48, 49] that indicated increased body dissatisfaction during pregnancy.

Conway *et al.* continued the research on restrictors and non-restrictors by assessing primigravid and primiparous women using the *Revised Restraint Scale (RRS)* in early pregnancy (n=62) [52]. They also completed *the Pregnancy and Weight Attitude Scale* later in pregnancy. In keeping with Restraint Theory[1], restrictive eaters had a higher pre-pregnancy BMI compared to non-restrictors [53-55]. As expected, restrictors had a

[1] Restraint theory (Heatherthon et al 1991, Herman and Polivy 1980, Herman and Mack 1975) proposes that restrained eaters may overeat and show disinhibitory eating in response to a range of triggers, many of which are characteristic of pregnancy.

significantly more negative attitude towards weight gain during pregnancy as evidenced by a lower average score on the PWGAS. There was no difference between the mean weight gain of the restrained and unrestrained eaters during pregnancy. However, when the women's weight gains were compared with recommendations at the time it was revealed that significantly fewer restrained eaters experienced weight gains within the recommended range for their pre-pregnancy BMI than did unrestrained eaters [52]. They mostly gained above or below the recommended guidelines. This group's characteristics and their experiences are similar to the group of past dieters in the previously described study by Fairburn and Welch [1]. In addition, Mela and Rogers suggested that repeated cycles of dieting and over-eating may distort restrained eaters' ability to perceive internal hunger and satiety cues [56] and thus may lead to higher or lower caloric intake. This literature highlights that pregravid levels of dietary restraint has an adverse effect on eating behaviour and unhealthy GWG during pregnancy, which is of considerable importance given unhealthy amounts of GWG are associated with greater health risks to mother and baby [15].

Fox and Yamaguchi assessed body image changes in pregnancy comparing normal weight and overweight women. They proposed that there may be a difference in attitudes between the two groups [57] and evaluated this using the 34-item *Body Shape Questionnaire.* Similar to the findings of Fairburn who showed that eating concerns decrease early in pregnancy but increase again as pregnancy progresses, [1] Fox and Yamaguchi noted that normal weight women reported less concern about their body image in the third trimester of pregnancy compared to overweight women. Additionally, they demonstrated that overweight women experienced an opposite shift with respect to perception of body image and reported a positive change in comparison to their pre-pregnancy body image [57] suggesting acceptability of extra weight when pregnant.

With the availability of research on this topic growing, by 1999, Baker and colleagues hypothesized that a woman's eating and weight concerns generally remain the same throughout pregnancy, but specific attitudes and behaviours change between pregnancy and post-partum [58]. They assessed women using both the *Eating Attitudes Test* (EAT), a 26-item self-report that identifies eating disturbances in a nonclinical population [43], and a *Satisfaction and Dieting* questionnaire that includes items about weight, dieting behaviour, and weight/shape satisfaction. Interestingly, an association between BMI and weight/shape satisfaction was noted suggesting that satisfaction is inversely related to actual weight. As previously reported in other studies, participants were more satisfied during pregnancy than at 4 months postpartum [58]. This highlights the need to monitor women not only during their pregnancy but postpartum as well as this represents an additional transition period of body image change linked to pregnancy.

The New Millennium: After 2000

Over the last decade, as maternal obesity has reached epidemic proportions, the body of work related to pregnancy behaviours, body image and weight gain attitudes has continued to grow. A prospective study which involved interviewing 19 women over the course of pregnancy identified that pregnant women adopt a pragmatic approach to weight gain and while they may be hesitant at first to accept the changes, most women will eventually recognize that this is only a temporary state [59]. These findings were similar to those of Davies and Wardle [51] who reported lower scores on *Drive for Thinness* subscale of the *Eating Disorder Inventory* for pregnant women and lower *Body Dissatisfaction Scale* scores compared to non-pregnant women. Around the same time, Boscaglia's group [60] was exploring the concept that exercise may have an impact on attitude towards body image by comparing results of the *Body Image Satisfaction* (BIS) questionnaire [61] from pre-pregnancy to the second trimester. For the high exercising group (baseline 251.25 ± 114.18 min/week), women were more satisfied with their bodies at 15-22 weeks gestation compared to 6 months pre-pregnancy. The high exercising group was also found to be significantly more satisfied with their bodies at 15-22 weeks gestation compared to the low exercising (baseline 39.03 ± 47.28 min/week) pregnant women. These findings suggest that regular exercise may enhance body image, particularly in the early phases of pregnancy. Exercise can also have a beneficial effect in regards to attitudes towards changes in specific body parts [61]. Of note, the majority of high exercisers attended group classes, which allowed the opportunity for social comparison with other pregnant women which may have contributed to differences in BIS between high and low exercisers [60]. The presence of other women alleviates the impact of the bodily changes; sharing personal experiences and seeing the same changes in other women may facilitate the acceptance of the pregnant state.

A recent study comparing obese to non-obese women found that before pregnancy the obese women had greater weight and shape concerns which then carried into pregnancy [62]. With regards to 'feeling fat', Duncombe et al., reported that satisfaction with body image was generally stable during the course of pregnancy, and, while participants in late pregnancy preferred a smaller belly, they did not feel as 'fat' as earlier in the pregnancy or during the pre-pregnancy period [63]. A previous qualitative study, which interviewed women during pregnancy, found that in the early phases of pregnancy, women felt 'fat' rather than pregnant because they were concerned that people may perceive them as such since it was not yet visually obvious that they were pregnant. While later in pregnancy as it becomes apparent that they are pregnant, and they felt comfortable with being identified as a pregnant woman, their weight and shape concerns were lessened [10]. These comments contrast studies with other qualitative studies that demonstrated a more positive attitude in the early phases of pregnancy and a decline in the last trimester [1]. Concerns about other people's attitude towards pregnant women have emerged as a contributor to body image and seem to play a role in women's attitudes towards their body. Clark et al. conducted in-depth, semi-structured interviews with 20 perinatal women (10 in late pregnancy, 10 in early postpartum). Two main themes emerged from the interviews regarding women's experience with their body during pregnancy. These themes were categorized as: 1) "I changed my body for baby, but that's OK" 2) "My social functioning has changed and I'm concerned about how people now perceive me". When asked about their feelings towards their body, half the women asserted that their decreased ability to exercise during pregnancy forced them to relax the amount of control they normally exerted over their body weight and shape through exercising. Although women expressed a concern on how they are being perceived, the pregnant state is often used as an excuse to eat more and exercise less [10].

In order to examine actual weight gain and perception of 'ideal' and current body sizes, Mehta and colleagues assessed 1,192 women using the BIA-O [64] at 15-20 weeks gestation [65]. The mean pre-gravid BMI in their population was 25.77 ± 6.88 kg/m^2. Sixty-four percent gained excessively during pregnancy and the mean adequacy of weight gain ratio (observed/expected weight gain) of 1.54 ± 0.83 indicates that women gained, on average, 54% more weight than expected. Women who preferred to be thinner were at higher risk of excessive weight gain compared to women who were happy with their body shape (i.e., their current body shape was not different from their 'ideal'). The risk associated with the desire to be thin decreased with increasing BMI; women who preferred to be heavier had an increased risk of gaining excessively as their pre-pregnancy BMI increased [65]. Women in the overweight and obese categories were at decreased risk of gaining excessively while women in the average and underweight BMI were at greater risk of excessive weight gain during pregnancy [65]. The authors suggested that women in the normal and underweight categories may experience a relaxation of pre-pregnancy body image ideals and become more comfortable with weight gain as their pregnancy progresses however, these results do not align with any current epidemiological data that have consistently shown women in the overweight and obese BMI categories tend to exceed GWG recommendations more often than not [29, 66-68].

Lastly, Loth and colleagues explored the responses of 995 female participants, of which 68 were pregnant, [69] on the *Body Shape Satisfaction Scale* [44]. In accordance with previous work, responses to this questionnaire assessing satisfaction with different body parts found that mean body satisfaction was significantly higher in pregnant than non-pregnant women. Although the association between pregnancy and *body satisfaction* differed for women who already had a child, secondary analysis indicated that *body satisfaction improvement* does not differ between primi- and multiparous women. Loth and colleagues suggested that in conjunction with previous research, there is something about the experience of being pregnant that increases a women's satisfaction with her physical appearance and indicates that despite the weight gain and physical changes that accompany pregnancy, women are able to navigate this transition in a positive way. The prospective nature of their study design allowed this group to examine a woman's body satisfaction prior to her pregnancy without concern that her current pregnancy might alter the way she remembered her former body satisfaction [69].

What We Know

A woman's ideals around body shape and weight may change during pregnancy. In general, pregnant women have a more positive attitude towards their body than non-pregnant women related to:

- acceptance of weight gain
- relaxation of weight-related psychological pressure; and
- shift from importance of body image perceptions towards health and wellbeing of the developing fetus

Perceptions of body image may differ from the start to end of pregnancy. Although not conclusive, in general, research has shown that women's attitudes transition from relatively positive to more negative over the course of pregnancy. This may be impacted by:

- *Pre-pregnancy weight*: there appears to be a positive association between pre-pregnancy body mass index and weight/shape satisfaction in pregnancy (i.e. body image satisfaction is closely tied to actual weight for overweight and obese women) [58]
- *Parity*: primiparous women tend to have fewer concerns about body image earlier in the pregnancy compared to later;
- *Diet history and eating behaviours*: past dieters are a high-risk group for both poor body image and the use of potentially harmful weight loss behaviours during pregnancy.

What Knowledge Gaps Exist?

To date, most of the research in this field has generally focused on weight gain in pregnancy and its effects on maternal and fetal physical health. Although there is an increasing amount of literature on maternal perceptions of this weight gain, body shape and body image, it is limited in several ways. For example, the existing literature is limited by numerous methodological issues: selection bias, recall bias, lack of proper comparison groups, and use of a single time point in pregnancy. Furthermore, the results may not be generalizable to contemporary cohorts of women as many of the studies were conducted 20-30 years ago prior to the dramatic rise in obesity rates. As such, future research needs to address these methodological limitations while focusing on maternal perceptions in order to better understand and develop targeted clinical interventions to address achieving healthy weight gain in the presence of adverse body image perceptions during pregnancy

Objective of This Chapter

The goal for this chapter is to provide an assessment body image, weight gain and associated attitudes towards weight gain during pregnancy using a prospective study that follows pregnant woman over the course of their pregnancy.

Using the ongoing Maternal Obesity Management (MOM) Trial (ISRCTN 75323409) [70], we are able to address many of the methodological limitations in the published literature in examining body weight and image in pregnancy.

Specifically we will look to:

I) Examine how the different factors, including women's attitudes, may affect weight gain and self-esteem (e.g. body image) in relation to maternal characteristics: parity, pre-pregnancy BMI (normal weight, overweight, obese) and gestational weight gain (adequate versus excessive);
II) Investigate temporal patterns in gestational weight gain and its associated eating-related attitudes across 3 times points in pregnancy; and
III) Assess adequacy of total gestational weight gain (GWG) between the pre-pregnancy BMI categories in relation the updated 2009 IOM guidelines.

Study Methods

Participants

Women from Ottawa, Canada were recruited at the end of their 1st trimester/beginning of their 2nd trimester (< 20 weeks gestation) through their health care provider (OB/GYN, family physician, mid-wife) or through advertisements. Normal weight, overweight, or obese pregnant women (pre-pregnancy BMI $\geq$ 18.5 kg/m^2) who were 18 years or older, known to be carrying a singleton fetus, with plans to deliver locally and keep the infant, were eligible for this trial. Women were excluded if they were smokers, had medical conditions that might impact body weight (e.g., pre-pregnancy insulin treated diabetes) or who have known contraindications to exercise as outlined in the joint SOGC/CSEP clinical practice guidelines [71].

Study Protocol

Three questionnaires (*pregnancy experience scale; pregnancy weight gain and attitude scale; diet history*), as described below, were used to investigate potential differences in GWG and attitudes towards weight during pregnancy. These questionnaires were administered at approximately 12-20 weeks (baseline/V1), 26-28 weeks (visit 2/V2) and >36 weeks (visit 3/V3) gestation. In addition, self-reported pre-pregnancy weight and height were collected, from which body mass index (BMI) and GWG were calculated. BMI was calculated according to the following formula: BMI=weight (kg)/height (m^2). Three different classifications of BMI were used: normal weight 18.5-24.9

kg/m^2; overweight 25-29.9 kg/m^2; obese ≥ 30+ kg/m^2. Demographic variables and participant characteristics were also collected on the participants including ethnicity, marital status, education, employment, total household income, age and parity.

The *pregnancy experience scale (PES)* is a validated questionnaire consisting of 41 items, with one specific question related to weight. Each question is based on two four-point Likert scales where each item is rated on the degree to which it is a hassle (negative) and/or an uplift (positive) from 0 “Not at all” to 3 “A great deal” [38]. Frequency (number of endorsed items) and intensity (sum of scores for endorsed items/number of endorsed items) were calculated for both the hassles and uplifts, where endorsed items refers to the items with a score greater than 0 [38]. Additionally, there is a composite ratio score (CRS) for frequency (frequency hassles/ frequency uplifts) and intensity (intensity hassles/ intensity uplifts) [38]. The pregnancy experience is considered to be more of a hassle if a CRS is greater than one and more of an uplift if a CRS is less than one [38]. This scale has displayed excellent internal consistency reliability (hassles: $\alpha = 0.95$; uplifts: $\alpha=0.91$) and good test-retest reliability correlations ($r = 0.56$ to 0.83). The test-retest reliability over the course of pregnancy in the present study was similar to previous reports ($r = 0.423 – 0.897$). Of note, the internal consistency reliability of the scale in our population over time was also similar to the original tests (hassles: $\alpha = 0.832 – 0.949$; uplifts: α=0.922-0.940).

The *pregnancy weight gain and attitude scale (PWGAS)* evaluates attitudes towards weight gain, physical appearance, and self-esteem to determine how these may affect actual weight gain during pregnancy [2]. It consists of 18 items with 15 questions related to weight and three related to behaviour [72]. Each response is rated on a four-point Likert scale from strongly agree to strongly disagree [72]. An average score is calculated for each participant based on all of the items in the scale; with an average score of three or greater indicating a positive attitude during pregnancy and less than three indicating a negative attitude [72]. There was moderate reliability in the original validation of this questionnaire using the split-half reliability method ($r=0.67$) [2]. This present study showed similar internal consistency reliability ($r = 0.663 – 0.824$) over the course of pregnancy as well as good test-retest reliability ($\alpha = 0.657$-0.788).

The *diet history questionnaire* is a standard questionnaire used in our research studies with women (pregnant or not) that assesses eating behaviours and dieting history prior to pregnancy to determine cyclic dieters (by number of times on a diet and lost more than 10 kg), restrictors (by number of times on a diet to lose weight in the last 5 years), disordered eating behaviours (by frequency of use of laxatives, diuretics, appetite control medication, binging and purging to control weight), as well as the age at first attempt to diet, and weight at 15, 25 and 35 years old to assess overall weight fluctuation. As this questionnaire is a reflection of past events it is only measured at the baseline visit.

Statistical Analyses

All results are presented as mean ± SEM. Statistical significance threshold was set at $p<0.05$, unless otherwise stated. All statistical analyses were performed using SPSS 20.0 (IBM, USA).

Analyses by Comparison Groups

To explore differences in attitudes towards weight gain, actual GWG and experiences during pregnancy, women were stratified into three pre-planned groups (known to influence these outcomes) for the following analyses:

i) Nulliparous vs. Primi/Multiparous
   - Nulliparous pregnant women were defined as those experiencing pregnancy for the first time and having no previous children as compared to primiparous or multiparous pregnant women who currently have 1 or more children at home
ii) Pre-pregnancy BMI (normal weight, overweight, obese)
   - Definitions for the three pre-pregnancy BMI categories as previously described in the study protocol section
iii) Adequate versus excessive gestational weight gain; these measures were adapted from Bondar et al. [73]
   - The assessment of adequate versus excessive GWG is based on the total weight gain at visit 3 (V3), during the last few weeks of the third trimester. An assumption of a 2.0 kg of weight gain in the first trimester is made for all pre-pregnancy BMI categories [27]. Expected total weight gain at the end of pregnancy for a normal weight woman is shown below. A similar calculation is performed for overweight and obese women by substituting 0.4 kg/week for 0.3 and 0.2 kg/week, respectively.

     Expected GWG = 2.0 kg + [(Gestational Age at V3 – 13 weeks) X 0.4 kg/week]

- The percentage range of expected weight gain is a ratio between the IOM guidelines for total gestational weight gain (per pre-pregnancy BMI category) to the gestational-age adjusted GWG, calculated above. For example, the IOM recommended GWG for normal women is 11.5 to 16 kg. Below are the formulas for minimum and maximum percentage gain. This procedure was replicated for overweight (7-11.5 kg) and obese (5-9 kg) women.

  Minimum percentage gain = (11.5 kg/expected weight gain) X 100
  Maximum percentage gain = (16 kg/expected weight gain) X 100

- For each individual participant, the adequacy of gestational weight gain is defined by the following formula:

  Adequacy of GWG = (Actual weight gain/Expected weight gain) X 100

  Participants are classified as having adequate gestational weight gain if their ratio of actual to expected weight gain falls within the minimum and maximum percentages of expected weight gain. Participants were classified as having excessive gestational weight gain if their ratio of actual to expected weight gain is higher than the maximum percentage of gestational weight gain.

For each of the three pre-planned groups, initial analysis involved comparing the demographic and individual level variables between the groups using Mann U Whitney non-parametric tests. Any related variables would be considered for possible inclusion as a covariate in further analyses. Specific procedures for each of comparison groups are described below.

Analysis by Measurement Scales

1. *Pregnancy Experience Scale (PES)*: square root transformations, reflections and reciprocal transformations were applied to PES measures prior to analysis where necessary. Linear mixture models with group as the independent factor, and time (V1-V3) as the repeated measure with a first-order autoregressive covariance matrix were used to investigate potential time and group differences in the

six main PES scales. Individual questionnaire items for uplifts and hassles from the PES at baseline only were analyzed using the Mann U Whitney non-parametric test for the nulli-and multiparous group and the gestational weight gain group. In the pre-pregnancy BMI group, individual questions from the PES at baseline only were analyzed using Kruskal Wallis non-parametric test with post hoc Mann U Whitney comparisons. Adjustment for multiple comparisons using a Bonferroni correction was performed; setting statistical significance threshold was set at $p<0.017$. Individual questions were also analyzed after adjusting for covariates using Quade's rank analysis of covariance [74].

2. *Pregnancy Weight Gain and Attitude Scale (PWGAS)*: Reciprocal transformation was applied to the mean PWGAS scores for the pre-pregnancy BMI comparison group prior to entering into the linear mixture model. Linear mixture models with group as the independent factor, and time (V1-V3) as the repeated measure with a first-order autoregressive covariance matrix were used to investigate potential time and group differences in the average score on the PWGAS for each of the three pre-planned groups. Individual questions from the PWGAS are analyzed using the same procedures from the PES.
3. *Diet History Questionnaire*: Procedures for analyzing individual questions were the same as used for the PES and PWGAS with the only exception that non-Likert items on this questionnaire were analyzed using independent samples t-test. Individual questions were also analyzed using the same procedures as PES and PWGAS.

Analyses by Clinical Outcomes

Gestational weight gain was evaluated between the pre-planned groups using linear mixture models with group as the independent factor, and time (V1-V3) as the repeated measure with a first-order autoregressive covariance matrix.

Post hoc analyses were performed for the pre-pregnancy BMI groups to determine potential differences between the three groups. Adjustment for multiple comparisons using a Bonferroni correction was performed; setting the statistical significance threshold at $p<0.006$.

Results

The study is ongoing. At present, 73 women consented to participate in this study, which contributed to the sample at baseline or visit 1 (V1). At visit 2 (V2), there were 53 women and by visit 3, 37 women. Of the 73 pregnant women measured at baseline, 76.7% were Caucasian, 82.2% were married, and 69.9% were university educated. Ninety-two percent of participants were currently employed and 55.6% listed their household income as greater than $100,000. The reduction in sample size is related to a subset of women not yet reaching V2 or V3 (n=18) and a subset of women lost to follow-up (n=18). There are no significant differences in sociodemographic factors between these groups of women, except for education. There was a significant difference in education level (U=503.0; p=0.034) such that 57.1% of women with incomplete data had a university education with 81.6% of women with complete data has the same level of education. Demographic and individual-level variable analyses yielded significant differences in employment (U=546.0; p=0.008), and age (U=396.5, p=0.003) between nulli- and primi/multiparous women. Primi/multiparous women were significantly older than nulliparous women. However, a larger percentage of nulliparous women listed being employed full-time as compared to primi/multiparous women. Pre-pregnancy BMI categories were significantly different in marital status ($\chi^2(2)$= 8.366; p=0.011) and education ($\chi^2(2)$=8.572; p=0.014). A larger portion of obese women were listed as being married (93.8%) as compared to normal weight (85.7%) and overweight (66.7%) women. Furthermore, all normal weight women listed as having a university-level education as compared to 55.6% of overweight women and 68.8% of obese women with the same level of education. Thus further analyses involving the nulli- and primi/multiparous groups as well as the pre-pregnancy BMI groups were adjusted for their potential confounding factors. There were no significant differences in any of the tested variables for the adequate versus excessive GWG categories.

Pregnancy Experience Scale (PES)

Parity

The number of items endorsed as an uplifting experience during pregnancy was significantly different over time (by trimester) ($F_{91.58,2}$=4.610; p=0.012) with both nulliparous (Adjusted - V1: 30.60 ± 1.64; V2: 31.28 ± 1.83; V3: 32.32 ± 2.30) and primi/multiparous women (Adjusted – V1: 29.96

± 1.67; V2: 30.66 ± 1.84; V3: 31.77 ± 2.33) having an increasing number of uplifting items across the pregnancy. However, the frequency of uplifting items did not significantly differ between the groups. The composite ratio score (intensity) was relatively stable over time with no significant differences over the pregnancy period for the overall cohort. However, nulliparous women on average had significantly lower scores overall as compared to primi/multiparous women (Adjusted: 0.68 ± 0.013 vs. 0.78 ± 0.015; $F_{73.68,1}$=6.791; p=0.011)

Pre-pregnancy BMI

The number of items endorsed as uplifts was significantly different over the pregnancy period ($F_{91.66,2}$=4.66; p=0.012) with increasing scores for normal weight women (Adjusted – V1: 32.31 ± 3.05; V2: 32.91 ± 3.24; V3: 33.77 ± 3.97) and overweight women (Adjusted – V1: 29.17 ± 1.74; V2: 29.86 ± 1.90; V3: 31.08 ± 2.34), and obese women (Adjusted – V1: 30.31 ± 1.75; V2: 30.98 ± 1.95; V3: 32.08 ± 2.44). However, these total scores did not significantly differ between the three pre-pregnancy BMI groups.

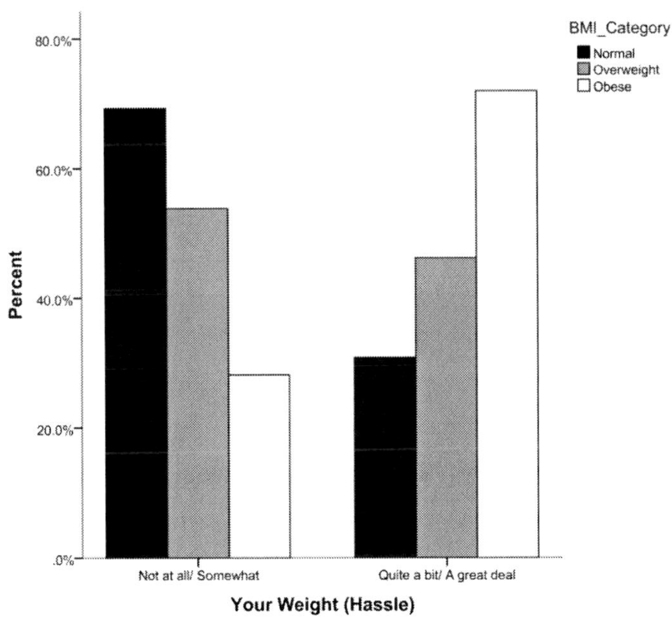

Figure 1. Percentage of respondents that rated weight to be a hassle on a rating scale from "Not at all/ Somewhat" to "Quite a bit/ A great deal", stratified by pre-pregnancy BMI category.

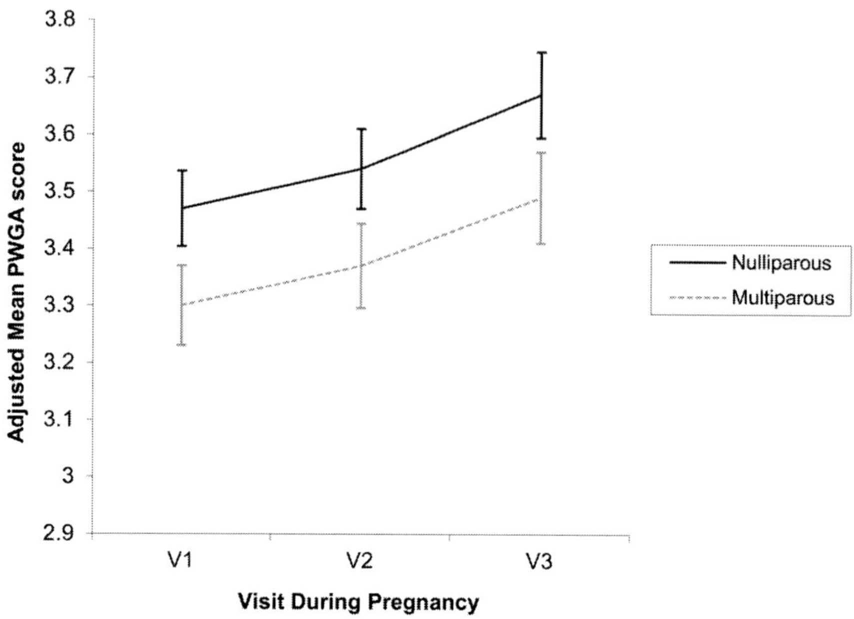

Figure 2. Mean PWGAS score over the course of pregnancy, stratified by parity. Error bars represent ± SEM. PWGAS, *Pregnancy Weight Gain and Attitude.*

When asked about their weight, 69.2% and 53.8% of normal and overweight women felt that their weight was "not at all" or "somewhat" of a hassle as compared to 71.9% of obese women felt that this was "quite a bit" or "a great deal" of a hassle ($\chi^2(2)= 7.479$; $p=0.022$). After conducting post-hoc analysis, it was identified that there were no significant differences in opinions between normal weight and obese women in regards to this issue (U=122.5; $p=0.018$) (Figure 1).

Adequate vs. Excessive GWG

There were no differences in the responses to the *Pregnancy Experience Scale* in those women who met versus exceeded the IOM GWG guidelines.

Pregnancy and Weight Gain Attitude Scale (PWGAS)

Parity

As Figure 2 indicates, the average adjusted PWGAS score increased significantly in nulli- and primi/multiparous women over the course of pregnancy suggesting an improvement in attitude [Nulliparous – V1: 3.47 ±

0.066; V2: 3.54 ± 0.070; V3: 3.67 ± 0.075, Multiparous – V1: 3.30 ± 0.070; V2: 3.37 ± 0.074; V3: 3.49 ± 0.080)($F_{89.17,2}$=6.095; p=0.003). However, the mean scores did not differ across parity groups.

Upon investigation of the individual questions on the PWGAS at baseline (V1), one question is particularly reflective of differing views between nulli- and primi/multiparous women. As shown in Figure 3, 69.2% of nulliparous women strongly disagree or disagree with the question "I am embarrassed at how big I have gotten during this pregnancy", while 29.4% of multiparous women were neutral in response to this question with a significant difference between the two groups (U=457.0; p=0.011). However after adjusting for the associated covariates, these differences were no longer significant ($F_{71,1}$=3.508; p=0.065).

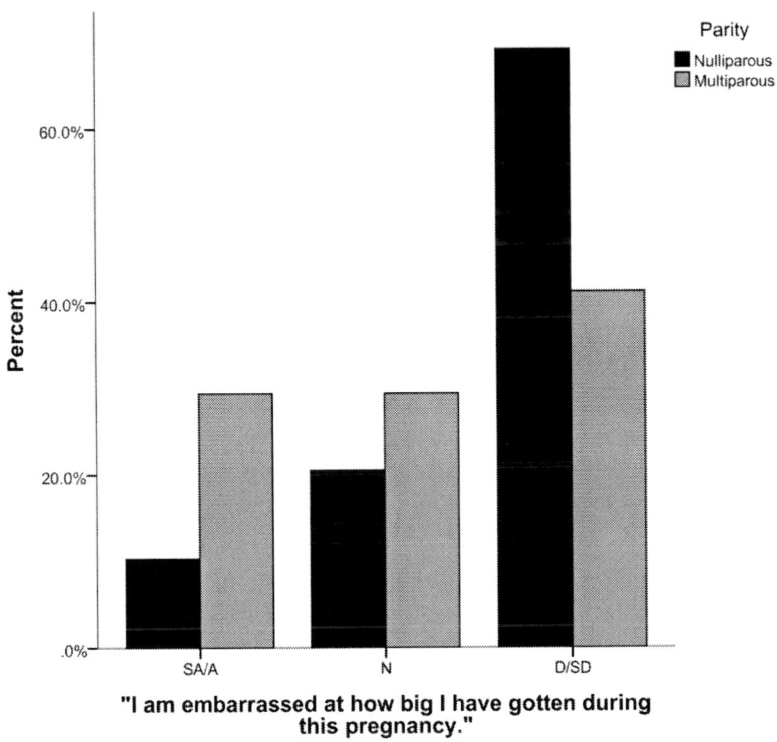

Figure 3. Distribution of respondents on a four-point Likert style question regarding body image from the *Pregnancy and Weight Gain Attitude Scale*, stratified by parity. Legend: SD= strongly disagree, D= disagree, N= neutral, A= agree, SA= strongly agree.

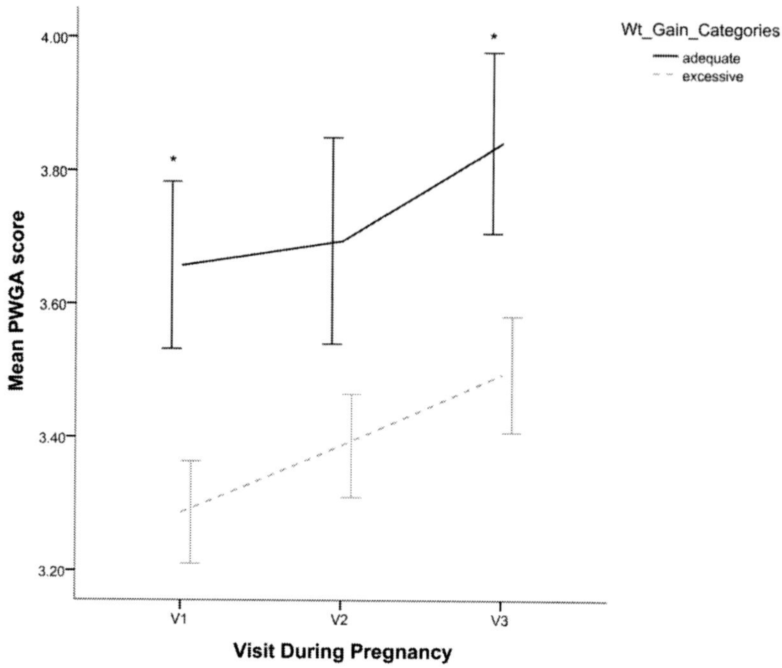

Figure 4. Mean PWGAS score over the course of pregnancy, stratified by gestational weight gain categories. Error bars represent ± SEM. *Legend:* PWGAS, *Pregnancy Weight Gain and Attitude. V1, visit 1; V2, visit 2; V3, visit 3.*

Pre-pregnancy BMI

Both normal weight and overweight women displayed attitudes that were comparable between V1 and V2 with a slightly higher score at the end of pregnancy (Adjusted – V1: 3.40 ± 0.11; V2: 3.47 ± 0.11; V3: 3.61 ± 0.13) and (Adjusted – V1: 3.32 ± 0.08; V2: 3.39 ± 0.08; V3: 3.52 ± 0.09) respectively. Obese women had steadily increasing positive attitudes scores over the course of pregnancy (Adjusted - V1: 3.28 ± 0.07; V2: 3.50 ± 0.10; V3: 3.62 ± 0.13) ($F_{89.71,2}$=5.020; p=0.009). However, when comparing across the three pre-pregnancy BMI groups, there were no significant differences in their PWGAS score over the course of pregnancy.

Adequate vs. Excessive GWG

As shown in Figure 4, women experiencing adequate or excessive weight gain both had increasing PWGAS scores over time, indicative of a significantly more positive attitude over time [Adequate (V1: 3.66 ± 0.13; V2: 3.70 ± 0.15; V3: 3.84 ± 0.14); Excessive (V1: 3.29 ± 0.08; V2: 3.39 ± 0.08;

V3: 3.50 ± 0.09)] ($F_{64.74,2}$=6.011; p=0.004). Women who gained an adequate amount of weight had overall higher scores than women that gained an excessive amount of weight with two significant time points over the course of pregnancy (3.73 ± 0.08 vs. 3.39 ± 0.05; $F_{32.96,1}$=7.128; *p*=0.012). There was no statistical interaction between the two different weight gain categories and time.

Diet History

Parity

There were no differences in the responses to any of the diet history questions in those women who are first time mothers versus those mothers that have other children at home.

Pre-pregnancy BMI

With respect to diet and weight, considering a particular event as the number of times that women have gone on a diet and lost more than 10 kgs, 84.6% of normal weight women have never experience such an event, 36.4% of overweight women have only experienced this event once, and 11.5% of obese women have experienced this event twice in their lifetime ($\chi^2(2)$= 15.391; *p*<0.0001). Overweight and obese women are more likely to report to have gone on a diet (once or twice) and lost 10 kg as compared to normal weight women (N-OW: U=73.5, *p*=0.009; N-OB: U=49.5, *p*<0.0001). These group differences remain statistically significant even after adjusting for the covariates ($F_{58,2}$=7.861; *p*=0.001).

Table 3. Diet History Information, stratified by BMI category

BMI category	Never Diet (%)[a]	Diet Once (%)[a]	Diet 2+ times (%)[a]	Age at first diet attempt (Mean ± SEM)	No. of times gone on a diet in 5 yrs
normal	84.6	7.7	7.7	15.63 ± 0.844	0.62 ± 0.311
overweight	36.4	36.4*	27.2	19.78 ± 1.315	1.93 ± 0.333
obese	19.2	26.9	46.0*	16.81 ± 0.882	1.76 ± 0.307

[a] In response to how many times in their lifetime they have gone on a diet and lost more than 10 kg.

* Overweight and obese women are significantly different than their normal weight comparators where the majority have never gone on a diet and lost more than 10 kg.

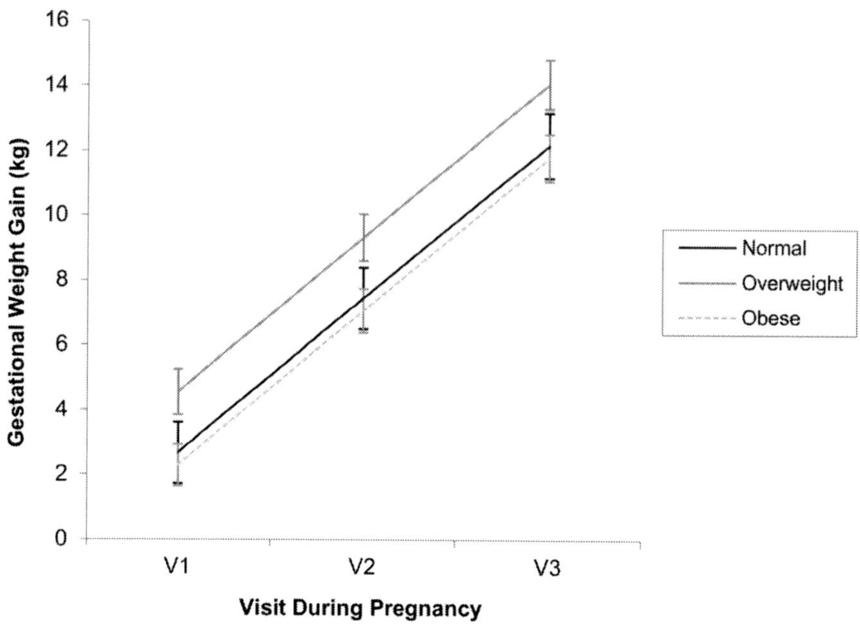

Figure 5. Gestational weight gain over the course of pregnancy as assessed by in three pre-pregnancy BMI categories: i) normal weight, ii) overweight; iii) obese. Legend: BMI, body mass index; V1, visit 1; V2, visit 2; V3, visit 3.

Reporting on the number of overall times that women in the pre-pregnancy BMI categories went on a diet in the past five years highlighted that 69.2% of normal weight women report having never been on a diet as compared to 20% of overweight and 16.0% of obese women that reported no history of dieting($\chi^2(2)$= 8.825; *p*=0.010). Significantly higher proportions of overweight and obese women have been on a diet at least once as compared to normal weight women (N-OW: U=62.000, p=0.008; N-OB: U=77.000, *p*=0.006). These values remain statistically significantly different after accounting for the covariates ($F_{55,2}$=5.078; *p*=0.009). Table 3 outlines key diet history findings.

Adequate vs. Excessive GWG

There were no differences in the responses to the diet history questionnaire in those women who met vs. exceeded the IOM GWG guidelines.

Table 4. Comparison of actual GWG to the recommend GWG guidelines from the Institute of Medicine (IOM) [27], stratified based on each of three pre-pregnancy BMI categories

	Average rate of gestational weight gain in the second and third trimesters of pregnancy		
Pre-pregnancy BMI Category	2nd Trimester (kg/week)	3rd Trimester (kg/week)	IOM guidelines (kg/week)
Normal Weight (BMI 18.5-24.9)	0.47 ± 0.03[a]	0.34 ± 0.06[b]	0.4
Overweight (BMI 25.0-29.9)	0.57 ± 0.04[c]	0.58 ± 0.05[d]	0.3
Obese (BMI > 30)	0.32 ± 0.04[e]	0.51 ± 0.06[f]	0.2

[a] n=11; [b] n=6; [c] n=19; [d] n=14; [e] n=19; [f] n=15.

Legend: BMI, Body mass index; IOM, Institutes of Medicine.

Note: The rate of weight gain in the 2nd trimester is calculated using GWG between V1 and V2 (~ second trimester) divided by the number of weeks between the V1 and V2. The rate of weight gain in the 3rd trimester is calculated using GWG between V2 and V3 (~ third trimester) divided by the number of weeks between the V2 and V3.

Gestational Weight Gain (GWG)

Pre-pregnancy BMI

As displayed in Figure 5, there was a significant increase in GWG over the three trimesters in all pre-pregnancy BMI categories (Adjusted NW: V1: 2.67 ± 0.95; V2: 7.44 ± 0.95; V3: 12.17 ± 1.00, Adjusted OW: V1: 4.55 ± 0.70; V2: 9.32 ± 0.72; V3: 14.06 ± 0.76, Adjusted OB: V1: 2.29 ± 0.64; V2: 7.06 ± 0.68; V3: 11.79 ± 0.72) ($F_{90.55,2}$=183.795; p <0.001). There was a significant difference between the three pre-pregnancy BMI groups in terms of their GWG ($F_{67.89,2}$=3.23; *p* = 0.046).

Over the duration of pregnancy, overweight women had significantly higher weight gain when compared to obese women ($t_{68.71}$=2.461; p <0.016). As shown in Table 4 both overweight and obese women exceeded the recommended rate of gestational weight gain for the second and third trimesters of pregnancy as set out by the IOM.

Interestingly, normal weight women slightly exceeded the recommendation in the second trimester but were within the guidelines in the third trimester.

Conclusion

We explored attitudes towards weight gain and body image prospectively based on *a priori* constructs known to influence weight gain and body image. The groups were stratified based on i) parity; ii) pre-pregnancy BMI; and iii) adequacy of weight gain. Analysis of individual and demographic variables exposed significant differences between nulli- and primi/multiparous women in terms of their overall age and employment. Primi/multiparous women were significantly older than nulliparous women. This might be expected as women who presently have children at home may represent further progression along their life course. Furthermore, all nulliparous women were employed compared to 82.4% of primi/multiparous women who were presently employed; highlighting the additional responsibilities of primi/multiparous women such as staying at home to raise other children. Marital status and education were found to differ between categories of pre-pregnancy BMI.

Parity

Our data from the PES indicate that as pregnancy progressed there was an increase in the number of uplifting items reported by both the nulli- and primi/multiparous groups, however the scores for the primi/multi group were slightly lower at each time point indicating that perhaps pregnancy is less of an uplifting experience for primi/multiparous women, having already previously experienced it. Similarly the composite score for intensity (intensity hassles/ intensity uplifts) for primi/multiparas was consistently lower than that of nulliparous women. While still considered a positive event overall, women who have previously experienced pregnancy and the associated weight gain-loss cycle, and who have additional children at home, may score certain items slightly less positively. Additionally, if the multiparous women did not return to their pre-pregnancy weight during the intra-partum period, then additional weight gain in subsequent pregnancies may be of greater concern and result in added stress.

Although primi/multiparous women's attitudes towards weight gain in pregnancy were not statistically different than their nulliparous comparators, their scores were lower at each time point. Analysis of our pregnant sample illustrated an increasing positive view over the course of pregnancy in both nulli- and primi/multiparous women as opposed to a stable view previously identified in the literature [63]. Early work in this area has reported a negative attitude in the last trimester compared to pre- and post-pregnancy [48, 49], although our study design did not lend itself to this examination.

Figure 3 depicts responses to the question related to whether or not a woman is embarrassed by the weight she has gained during pregnancy. Our results display that a greater percentage of nulliparous women are not embarrassed by the weight gain, which may indicate a certain a degree of pride during their pregnancy- a novelty that may not be there for those who have experienced this before. However, after adjusting for age and employment, these effects are no longer significant suggesting that sociodemographic factors influence how women feel about their weight gain during pregnancy and thus evaluate their current situation.

BMI Category

Exploring the experience of pregnancy in women of differing pre-gravid BMI we found that the frequency of endorsed uplifts increased over the course of pregnancy for all groups with the normal weight women reporting higher scores, overweight women reporting lower scores at each time point and obese women falling in between. Interestingly, we hypothesized that obese women would have the lowest score in terms of the frequency of endorsed uplifts and would be the least satisfied with the changes during pregnancy. However our data does not fully support this as obese women appear to be more accepting overall of the changes associated with pregnancy as compared to overweight women. However, one of the PES questions posed to women relates to whether or not weight was considered a hassle and as Figure 1 illustrates, there is an evident pattern in responses with obese women believing weight to be more of a hassle. But like many other comparisons that were made, after adjusting for covariates the difference was found to be non-significant.

Although there were no statistically significant differences between PWGAS pre-pregnancy BMI groups, normal weight women and overweight women reported relatively stable scores with a slightly 'better' attitude at the end of pregnancy. Obese women's scores increased throughout pregnancy but were slightly lower at the beginning and end of pregnancy when compared to their normal weight and overweight comparators. These results support the findings of Micali et al. who reported that obese women had greater body image concerns prior to and during pregnancy [71] and others who have suggested that women with high pre-pregnancy BMIs may already be concerned with their weight prior to pregnancy - a view that may carry through into pregnancy [62].

Adequate vs. Excessive GWG

Although we had predicted that women who exceeded weight gain guidelines would report a greater number or intensity of hassles on the PES, our data indicate that this was not the case since no differences were identified. Our data did demonstrate that women who gained weight within their recommended range had a significantly more positive attitude as reported by a higher PWGAS score compared to women who gained excessive gestational weight. This is in keeping with work by Skouteris *et al.* who reported that the psychological correlates of excessive GWG included greater body image dissatisfaction [75].

Diet History

While there were no differences in diet history between parity groups, our hypothesis that overweight or obese pregnant women would have a stronger dieting history than those of normal weight was confirmed by our data. However, the majority of normal weight women reported never having dieted to lose 10kg or more, which was significantly different from the overweight and obese women.

We had predicted that women who gained excessively may have had a robust history of dieting. Our hypothesis was based on the literature that has demonstrated an easing of restrictive eating behaviours during pregnancy (13), however we were surprised to observe no relationship between diet history and exceeding GWG guidelines in our sample. While we had hoped to examine the potential differences in PWGAS in regular dieters vs. non-dieters, our *a priori* 'dieter' criteria (1 diet attempt per year) identified only 3 women thus due to a small sample size, statistical analyses were not performed.

General Gestational Weight Gain

According to the mean data at visit 3 in the last few weeks (days) of pregnancy, both the overweight and obese groups had exceeded their GWG recommendation while the normal weight women were within their target range. It is not unusual for overweight or obese women to exceed the guidelines as their recommended weight gain range is much lower than for women who enter pregnancy at a normal weight [29, 68]. When looking at the rate of weight gain it is notable that rate of weight gain fell between the 2nd to the 3rd trimester to meet guidelines in normal weight women, while the rate was well over expected for overweight women and rose considerably over time in the obese women.

Strength and Limitations

Our analyses provide a novel longitudinal view of body image attitudes and influences towards weight gain across the entire duration of pregnancy while monitoring and adjusting for gestational weight gain. Unfortunately, our small sample at post-baseline assessments attributed to loss to follow-up, drop-out or having not yet reached assessment time point may limit generalization to the general pregnant population. On a positive note, the questionnaires utilized in this study had strong psychometric properties, thus indicating a high level of internal validity of the findings. While we were unable to assess all aspects of psychosocial health, the following scales have been designed for and have shown strong psychometric properties in pregnant women including the *Pregnancy Experience Scale* [38], *Maternal Social Support Index* [76], *The Edinburgh Postnatal Depression Scale* [77], and the *Pregnancy and Weight Gain Attitude Scale* [2]. In this chapter we focused on the two most relevant to body image and weight gain attitudes.

Future Directions

While this study primarily focused on the pregnancy period, future research is warranted to incorporate the post-partum period into the longitudinal analysis. Previous studies have shown that women are more satisfied during the pregnancy period than they are at 4 months postpartum [58]. Thus it would be important to investigate the validity of this finding in our population as well. It is also essential to examine the degree to which body image dissatisfaction and attitudes towards weight gain are triggered by women's current view of self and the degree to which these feelings are triggered by future thoughts of their body image during the postpartum period.

Assessing the exercise habits of pregnant women is also of interest, as exercise has been found to be associated with a more positive body image in the general population [78-80]. Although only a few studies have examined the association between exercise and body image in pregnant women [61, 81, 82] results suggest a trend toward a perception of enhanced body image with increased exercise.

Future studies in this area may wish to use additional questionnaires to further investigate different components of body image attitudes and weight gain. Such validated questionnaires as the *Revised Restraint Scale* (RRS) [52], Dutch Eating Behaviour Questionnaire [46], The Three Factor Eating Questionnaire [47], or *the Eating Attitudes Test* (EAT) [43, 83] would allow information on a broader scope of eating behaviour to tie in with attitudes towards weight.

Overall, examining body image and how it relates to eating behaviour and weight gain in pregnancy is a clinically relevant discussion topic and important area of research. These factors influence maternal perceptions, well-being and potential engagement in behaviours including healthy dietary intake and physical activity during pregnancy which are known to have a positive influence on the health of mom and baby. Practically speaking, health care providers who care for pregnant women should be aware that meeting gestational weight gain guidelines is important for not only physiological health but for a woman's emotional well-being as well.

References

[1] Fairburn C. G, Welch S. L. The Impact of Pregnancy on Eating Habits and Attitudes to Shape and Weight. *International Journal of Eating Disorders* 1990; 9 (2): 153-60.

[2] Palmer J. L, Jennings G. E, Massey L. Development of an assessment form: Attitude toward weight gain during pregnancy. *Journal of The American Dietetic Association* 1985; 85 (8): 946-9.

[3] Drake R, Cullum A. Don't ignore weight gain during pregnancy. *Br. J. Midwifery* 1998; 6: 211-4.

[4] Cash T. F. Body image: past, present, and future. *Body Image* 2004; 1: 1-5.

[5] Conti J, Abraham S, Taylor A. Eating behavior and pregnancy outcome. *J. Psychosom. Res.* 1998; 44 (3-4): 465-77.

[6] Bulik C. M, Sullivan P. F, Fear J. L, Pickering A, Dawn A, McCullin M. Fertility and reproduction in women with anorexia nervosa: a controlled study. *J. Clin. Psychiatry* 1999; 60 (2): 130-5.

[7] Franko D. L, Walton B. E. Pregnancy and eating disorders: a review and clinical implications. *Int. J. Eat. Disord.* 1993; 13 (1): 41-7.

[8] Shearer M. H. Malnutrition in middle class pregnant women. *Birth Fam. J.* 1980; 7: 27-35.

[9] Richardson P. Women's experiences of body change during normal pregnancy. *Matern. Child Nurs. J.* 1990; 19 (2): 93-111.

[10] Clark A, Skouteris H, Wertheim E. H, Paxton S. J, Milgrom J. A baby body: A qualitative insight into women's body-related experiences and mood during pregnancy and the postpartum. *Journal of Reproductive and Infant Psychology* 2009; 27 (4): 330-45.

[11] Wiles R. 'I'm not fat, I'm pregnant.' The impact of pregnancy on fat women's body language. *Health Psychol Update* 1993; 12: 16-21.

[12] Mumford S. L, Siega-Riz A. M, Herring A, Evenson K. R. Dietary restraint and gestational weight gain. J Am Diet Assoc 2008; 108 (10): 1646-53.

[13] Clark M, Ogden J. The impact of pregnancy on eating behaviour and aspects of weight concern. *International Journal of Obesity* 1999; 23: 18-24.

[14] Fairburn C. G, Stein A, Jones R. Eating Habits and Eating Disorders During Pregnancy. *Psychosomatic Medicine* 1992; 54: 665-72.

[15] Adamo K. B, Ferraro Z. M, Brett K. E. Can We Modify the Intrauterine Environment to Halt the Intergenerational Cycle of Obesity? *Int. J. Environ. Res. Public Health* 2012; 9: 1263-307.

[16] Wrotniak B. H, Shults J, Butts S, Stettler N. Gestational weight gain and risk of overweight in the offspring at age 7 y in a multicenter, multiethnic cohort study. *Am. J. Clin. Nutr.* 2008; 87 (6): 1818-24.

[17] Stevens-Simon C., McAnarney E. R. Determinants of weight gain in pregnant adolescents. *J. Am. Diet. Assoc.* 1992; 92 (11): 1348-51.

[18] Ekblad U, Grenman S. Maternal weight, weight gain during pregnancy and pregnancy outcome. *Int. J. Gynaecol. Obstet.* 1992; 39 (4): 277-83.

[19] Cedergren M. Effects of gestational weight gain and body mass index on obstetric outcome in Sweden. *Int. J. Gynaecol. Obstet.* 2006; 93 (3): 269-74.

[20] Catalano P. M, Ehrenberg H. M. The short- and long-term implications of maternal obesity on the mother and her offspring. *BJOG* 2006; 113 (10): 1126-33.

[21] Moreira P, Padez C, Mourão-Carvalhal I, Rosado V. Maternal weight gain during pregnancy and overweight in Portuguese children. *Int. J. Obes.* (Lond) 2007; 31 (4): 608-14.

[22] Oken E, Taveras E. M, Kleinman K. P, Rich-Edwards J. W, Gillman M. W. Gestational weight gain and child adiposity at age 3 years. *Am. J. Obstet. Gynecol.* 2007; 196 (4): 332e1-8.

[23] Stuebe A. M, Forman M. R, Michels K. B. Maternal-recalled gestational weight gain, pre-pregnancy body mass index, and obesity in the daughter. *Int. J. Obes.* (Lond) 2009; 33 (7): 743-52.

[24] Kim S. Y, Dietz P. M, England L, Morrow B, Callaghan W. M. Trends in pre-pregnancy obesity in nine states, 1993-2003. *Obesity* (Silver Spring) 2007; 15 (4): 986-93.

[25] Robinson H. E, O'Connell C. M, Joseph K. S, McLeod N. L. Maternal outcomes in pregnancies complicated by obesity. *Obstetrics and Gynecology* 2005; 106 (6): 1357-64.

[26] Hedley A. A, Ogden C. L, Johnson C. L, Carroll M. D, Curtin L. R, Flegal K. M. Prevalence of overweight and obesity among US children, adolescents, and adults, 1999-2002. *JAMA* 2004; 291 (23): 2847-50.

[27] Institute of Medicine, National Research Council. Weight Gain During Pregnancy: Reexamining the Guidelines. Washington, DC: The National Academies Press; 2009.

[28] Viswanathan M, Siega-Riz A. M, Moos M. K, Deierlein A, Mumford S, Knaack J, et al. Outcomes of maternal weight gain. *Evid. Rep. Technol. Assess.* (Full Rep) 2008; 168: 1-223.

[29] Ferraro Z. M, Barrowman N, Prud'homme D, Walker M, Wen S. W, Rodger M, et al. Excessive gestational weight gain predicts large for gestational age neonates independent of maternal body index. *J. Matern. Fetal Neonatal Med.* 2012; 25 (5): 538-42.

[30] Sebire N. J, Jolly M, Harris J. P, Wadsworth J, Joffe M, Beard R. W, et al. Maternal obesity and pregnancy outcome: a study of 287,213 pregnancies in London. *Int. J. Obes. Relat. Metab. Disord.* 2001; 25 (8): 1175-82.

[31] Rudra C. B, Williams M. A, Lee I. M, Miller R. S, Sorensen T. K. Perceived exertion during pre-pregnancy physical activity and preeclampsia risk. *Med. Sci. Sports Exerc.* 2013; 37 (11): 1836-41.

[32] O'Brien T. E, Ray J. G, Chan W. S. Maternal body mass index and the risk of preeclampsia: a systematic overview. *Epidemiology* 2003; 14 (3): 368-74.

[33] Nucci L. B, Schmidt M. I, Duncan B. B, Fuchs S. C, Fleck E. T, Santos Britto M. M. Nutritional status of pregnanct women: prevalence and associated pregnancy outcomes. *Rev. Saude Publica* 2001; 35 (6): 502-7.
[34] Frederick I. O, Rudra C. B, Miller R. S, Foster J. C, Williams M. A. Adult weight change, weight cycling, and pre-pregnancy obesity in relation to risk of preeclampsia. *Epidemiology* 2006; 17 (4): 428-34.
[35] Callaway L. K, Prins J. B, Chang A. M, McIntyre H. D. The prevalence and impact of overweight and obesity in an Australian obstetric population. *Med. J. Aust.* 2006; 184 (2): 56-9.
[36] Cooper Z, Fairburn C. G. The Eating Disorder Examination: A semi-structured interview for the assessment of the specific psychopathology of eating disorders. *Int. J. Eat. Disord.* 1987; 6: 1-8.
[37] Thompson J. K. Assessing body image disturbance: measures, methodology, and implementation. In: Thompson JK, editor. *Body image, eating disorders, and obesity: an integrative guide for assessment and treatment.* Washington, D.C.: American Psychological Association; 1996. p. 49-82.
[38] DiPietro J. A, Ghera M. M, Costigan K, Hawkins M. Measuring the ups and downs of pregnancy stress. *J. Psychosom. Obstet. Gynecol.* 2004; 25: 189-201.
[39] DeLongis A, Folkman S, Lazarus R. S. The impact of daily stress on health and mood: Psychological and social resources as mediators. *J. Pers. Soc. Psychol.* 1988; 54: 486-9.
[40] Cooper P, Taylor M, Cooper Z, Fairburn C. The development and validation of the body shape questionnaire. *Int. J. Eating Disorders* 1987; 6 (485): 494.
[41] Secord P. F, Jourard S. M. The appraisal of body-cathexis: body-cathexis and the self. *J. Consult. Psychol.* 1953; 17 (5): 343-7.
[42] Mirucka B. Kwestionariusz Ja Cielesnego (Skala J-C) [The Body Image Questionnaire]. *Przeglad Psychologiczny* [Review of Psychology] 2005; 48 (3): 313-29.
[43] Garner D. M, Garfinkel P. E. The Eating Attitudes Test: an index of the symptons of anorexia nervosa. *Psychol. Med.* 1979; 9 (2): 273-9.
[44] Pingitore R, Spring B, Garfield D. Gender differences in body satisfaction. *Obes. Res.* 1997; 5 (5): 402-9.
[45] Williamson D. A, Womble L. G, Zucker N. L, Reas D. L, White M. A, Blouin DC, et al. Body image assessment for obesity (BIA-O): Development of a new procedure. *International Journal of Obesity and Related Metabolic Disorders* 2000; 24 (10): 1326-32.

[46] van Strien T, Frijters J. E. R, Bergers G. P. A, Defares P. B. The Dutch Eatng Behavior Questionnaire (DEBQ) for assessment of restrained, emotional, and external eating behavior. *International Journal of Eating Disorders* 1986; 5 (2): 295-315.

[47] Stunkard A. J, Messick S. The three-factor eating questionnaire to measure dietary restraint, disinhibition and hunger. *Journal of Psychosomatic Research* 1985; 29 (1): 71-83.

[48] Slade P. D. Awareness of body dimensions during pregnancy: an analogue study. *Psychol. Med.* 1977; 7 (2): 245-52.

[49] Strang V. R, Sullivan P. L. Body Image Attitudes During Pregnancy and the Postpartum Period. *JOGNN* 1985; 332-7.

[50] Abraham S, King W, Llewellyn-Jones D. Attitudes to body weight, weight gain and eating behavior in pregnancy. *J. Psychosom. Obstet. Gynecol.* 1994; 15: 189-1995.

[51] Davies K, Wardle J. Body Image and Dieting in Pregnancy. *Journal of Psychosomatic Research* 1994; 38 (8): 787-99.

[52] Conway R, Reddy S, Davies J. Dietary restraint and weight gain during pregnancy. *European Journal of Clinical Nutrition* 1999; 53: 849-53.

[53] Herman C. P, Mack D. Restrained and unrestrained eatin. *J. Pers* 1975; 43 (4): 647-60.

[54] Heatherton T. F, Polivy J, Herman C. P. Restraint, weight loss, and variability of body weight. *J. Abnorm. Psychol.* 1991; 100 (1): 78-83.

[55] Herman C. P, Polivy J. *Restrained eating.* In: Stunkard A. J, editor. Obesity. Philadelphia, P.A.: Saunders; 1980. p. 208-25.

[56] Mela J, Rogers P. J. *Food, Eating and Obesity: The Psychobiological Basis of Appetite and Weight Control.* London: Chapman and Hall; 1998.

[57] Fox P, Yamaguchi C. Body Image Change in Pregnancy: A Comparison of Normal Weight and Overweight Primigravidas. *BIRTH* 1997; 24: 35-40.

[58] Baker C. W, Carter A. S, Cohen L. R, Brownell K. D. Eating Attitudes and Behaviors in Pregnancy and Postpartum: Global Stability versus Specific Transitions. *Ann. Behav. Med.* 1999; 21 (2): 143-8.

[59] Earle S. 'Bumps and boobs': Fatness and women's experience of pregnancy. *Women's Studies International Forum* 2003; 26: 245-52.

[60] Boscaglia N, Skouteris H, Wertheim E. H. Changes in body image satisfaction during pregnancy: A comparison of high exercising and low exercising women. *Australian and New Zealand Journal of Obstetrics and Gynaecology* 2003; 43: 41-5.

[61] Goodwin A, Astbury J, McMeekan J. Body image and psychological well-being in pregnancy. A comparison of exercisers and non-exercisers. *Australian and New Zealand Journal of Obstetrics and Gynaecology* 2000; 40 (4): 442-7.

[62] Micali N, Treasure J, Simonoff E. Eating disorders symptoms in pregnancy: a longitudinal study of women with recent and past eating disorders and obesity. *J. Psychosom. Res.* 2007; 63 (3): 297-303.

[63] Duncombe D, Wertheim E. H, Skouteris H, Paxton S. J, Kelly L. How Well Do Women Adapt to Changes in Their Body Size and Shape across the Course of Pregnancy? *J. Health Psychol.* 2008; 13: 503-15.

[64] Williamson D. A, Womble L. G, Zucker N. L, Reas D. L, White M. A, Blouin D. C, et al. Body image assessment for obesity (BIA-O): development of a new procedure. *Int. J. Obes. Relat. Metab. Disord.* 2000; 24 (10): 1326-32.

[65] Mehta U. J, Siega-Riz A. M, Herring A. H. Effect of Body Image on Pregnancy Weight Gain. *Matern. Child Health J.* 2011; 15: 324-32.

[66] Lowell H, Miller D. C. Weight gain during pregnancy: Adherence to Health Canada's guidelines. *Health Reports* 2010; 21: 31-6.

[67] Stotland N. E, Haas J. S, Brawarsky P, Jackson R. A, Fuentes-Afflick E, Escobar G. J. Body mass index, provider advice, and target gestational weight gain. *Obstetrics and Gynecology* 2005; 105: 633-8.

[68] Weisman C. S, Hillemeier M. M, Downs D. S, Chuang C. H, Dyer A. M. Preconception predictors of weight gain during pregnancy: Prospective findings from the Central Pennsylvania Women's Health Study. *Womens Health Issues* 2010; 20: 126-32.

[69] Loth K. A, Bauer K. W, Wall M, Berge J, Neumark-Sztainer D. Body satisfaction during pregnancy. *Body Image* 2011; 8: 297-300.

[70] Adamo K. B, Ferraro Z. M, Goldfield G. S, Keely E, Stacey D, Hadjiyannakis S, et al. The Maternal Obesity Management (MOM) Trial Protocol: A lifestyle intervention during pregnancy to minimize downstream obesity. *Contemporary Clinical Trials.* 2013; 35: 87-96.

[71] Davies G. A, Wolfe L. A, Mottola M. F, MacKinnon C. Joint SOGC/CSEP clinical practive guideline: Exercise in pregnancy and the postpartum period. *Can. J. Appl. Physiol.* 2003; 28: 330-41.

[72] DiPietro J. A, Millet S, Costigan K. A, Gurewitsch E, Caulfield L. E. Psychosocial influences on weight gain attitudes and behaviors during pregnancy. *J. Am. Diet Assoc.* 2003; 103: 1314-9.

[73] Bondar L. M, Siega-Riz A. M, Arab L, Chantala K, McDonald T. Predictors of pregnancy and postpartum haemoglobin concentrations in low-income women. *Public Health Nutrition* 2004; 7 (6): 701-11.

[74] Quade D. Rank analysis of covariance. *Journal of American Statistical Association* 1967; 62 (320): 1187-200.

[75] Skouteris H. Pregnancy: Physical and Body Image Changes. *Encyclopedia of Body Image and Human Appearance* 2012; 2: 664-8.

[76] Pascoe J. M, Ialongo N. S, Horn W. F, Reinhart M. A, Perradatto D. The reliability and validity of the maternal social support index. *Fam. Med.* 1988; 20 (4): 271-6.

[77] Cox J. L, Holden J. M, Sagovsky R. Development of the 10-item Edinburgh Postnatal Depression Scale. *Br. J. Psychiatry* 1987; 150: 782-6.

[78] Fisher E, Thompson J. K. A comparative evaluation of cognitive behavioral therapy (CBT) versus exercise therapy (ET) for the treatment of body image disturbance: Preliminary findings. *Behav. Modif.* 1994; 18: 171-85.

[79] Koniak-Griffin D. Aerobic exercise, psychological well-being, and physical discomforts during adolescent pregnancy. *Res. Nurs. Health* 1994; 17: 253-63.

[80] Kostanski M, Gullone E. Adolescent body image dissatisfaction: relationships with self-esteem, anxiety, and depression controlling for body mass. *J. Child Psychol. Psychiatry* 1998; 39: 255-62.

[81] Marquez-Sterling S, Perry A. C, Kaplan T. A, Halberstein R. A, Signorile J. F. Physical and psychological changes with vigorous exercise in sedentary primigravidae. *Med. Sci. Sports Exerc.* 2000; 32: 58-62.

[82] Walker L. O. Weight-related distress in the early months after childbirth. *West J. Nurs. Res.* 1998; 20: 30-44.

[83] Garner D. M, Olmstead M. P, Bohr Y, Garfinkel P. E. The eating attitudes test: psychometric features and clinical correlates. *Psychol. Med.* 1982; 12 (4): 871-88.

This chapter was reviewed by:

Becky Blair RD, MSc
Public Health Nutritionist,
Family Health Service Simcoe Muskoka District Health Unit,
Ontario Canada

Nicole Obeid PhD- Clin Psych
Inpatient Mental Health Research Group
Children's Hospital of Eastern Ontario
Ottawa, Ontario CAN

Marisa Murray MSc, PhD (c)
Department of Psychology
University of Ottawa
Ontario, CAN

In: Weight Gain
Editors: A. Pirotte and T. Libert

ISBN: 978-1-62618-800-6

Chapter 2

MATERNAL WEIGHT GAIN AND PERINATAL OUTCOMES

Hiroko Watanabe[1,*], Takashi Sugiyama[2] and Kwok-Kei Mak[3]

[1]Department of Clinical Nursing, Division of Maternity Nursing, Shiga University of Medical Science, Shiga, Japan

[2]Department of Gynecology and Obstetrics, Tohoku University Graduate School of Medicine, Miyagi, Japan

[3]Department of Community Medicine and School of Public Health, Faculty of Medicine, University of Hong Kong, Hong Kong

ABSTRACT

Weight gain management before and during pregnancy may be a key factor influencing the health of women during pregnancy and the development of the fetus. Adequate gestational weight gain contributes to better pregnancy outcomes in both mothers and infants, in short- and long-term. The Institute of Medicine (IOM) released gestational weight guidelines for optimal pregnancy outcomes. The guideline will be used in clinical practices for effective weight management aiming at improving fetal and maternal outcomes.

* Corresponding author: Hiroko Watanabe, Address; Seta Tsukinowa-cho, Otsu, Shiga, 520-2192, Japan. Tel: +81-77-548-2433. Fax: +81-77-548-2433. E-mail: watana@belle.shiga-med.ac.jp.

Evidences from human and animal studies of pre-pregnancy body mass index and gestational weight gain showed that altering the environment of utero could lead to lifelong health consequences, such as high adiposity, sarcopenia, insulin resistance, glucose intolerance, and high blood pressure. Population-based prospective cohort studies starting from different geographical regions in the pre-conceptional period or in early fetal life, in which the offspring is followed from early fetal life until young adulthood. All women of reproductive age are encouraged to follow the IOM recommendations and maintain a well-balanced diet. To improve birth outcomes, it is critical for women to modify their health behaviors for a better nutritional status before, during, and after conception.

Introduction

Pre-pregnancy body mass index (BMI) [weight (kg)/ height (m) ^{2}] and gestational weight gain (GWG) show a strong association with pregnancy outcomes. Low pre-pregnancy BMI is a strong predictor of preterm birth and fetal growth restriction [1, 2]. Previous reports also indicate that a normal pre--pregnancy BMI recommended weight gain is good for maternal and newborn health [3, 4]. During pregnancy, obese pregnant women may develop peripheral and hepatic insulin resistance, which could lead to gestational diabetes [5]. Adequate gestational weight gain contributes to better short- and long-term health outcomes of both mothers and infants. On the other hand, recent research suggests that inadequate levels of maternal nutrients during the crucial period of fetal development may lead to reprogramming within the fetal tissues that predisposes the infant to chronic illnesses in adulthood [6-8]. However, many women of childbearing age do not maintain a healthy diet before conception or during pregnancy. Laraia et al. [9] found that pre-pregnancy weight status is associated with diet quality during pregnancy and the subsequent gestational weight status. Women who were pre-conceptionally overweight are 7.4 times more likely to gain excessive weight during pregnancy [10].

The adoption of the Institute of Medicine's (IOM) new recommendations [11] for pregnancy weight gain in pregnant women, especially for obese and overweight groups, is encouraged to improve their pregnancy outcomes. A better understanding of the influences of maternal weight gain management on women's health during pregnancy and fetal development is warranted for clinical practices.

CURRENT ISSUES OF REPRODUCTIVE WOMEN'S BODY COMPOSITIONS

BMI is generally accepted as a good anthropometric indicator of overall adult nutritional status and body fat. The World Health Organization defines underweight as a BMI of less than 18.5, normal weight as a BMI of 18.5–24.9, overweight as a BMI of 25–29.9, and obesity as a BMI of 30 or greater [12]. Obesity is further characterized by BMI into class I (30 –34.9), class II (35–39.9), and class III (greater than 40) [12].

There is a great concern of high prevalence and increasing trend of obesity worldwide, especially in Western societies. In the National Health and Nutrition Examination Survey (NHANES), the prevalence of obesity (BMI $\geq$30 kg/m^2) in women aged 20-39 years continues to be high, exceeding 30% after 2005 (Figure 1) [13].

In the latest NHANES data from 2009-2010 in women at the age 20-39 years, the prevalence of overweight (BMI $\geq$25 kg/m^2) and obesity were 55.8% and 31.9%, respectively. The prevalence was highest among low income black, Hispanic, and white women in the United States [13]. Similar trends are observed in other developed countries.

Maternal size before conception plays a key role in determining perinatal outcomes (Table 1). A pre-pregnancy BMI within the normal range is important to maintain maternal health during and after pregnancy. In women of reproductive age, high pre-pregnancy BMI, i.e., overweight and obesity, is associated with infertility and increased risk of miscarriage [14, 15]. During pregnancy, obesity is a risk factor for adverse pregnancy outcomes such as gestational diabetes, preeclampsia, cesarean delivery, and complications at delivery [16, 17].

In the UK, more than 50% of women in the reproductive age group (25-44 years) are overweight or obese. Over 15 years, from 1990 to 2004, there has been a 69% increase in maternal obesity [18]. In Australia in 2007-2008, 44.5% women at age 25-34 years and 55.3% women at age 35-44 years are overweight or obese, which constitutes a marked increase over the last 20 years [19]. Therefore, increase in obesity in reproductive age women is a worldwide phenomenon. This increasing trends of obesity is attributable to a combination of reduced exercise, changing dietary composition, and increased caloric intake.

In addition to obesity, the increasing trends of underweight (BMI<18.5 kg/m^2) are also a risk factor for adverse pregnancy outcomes.

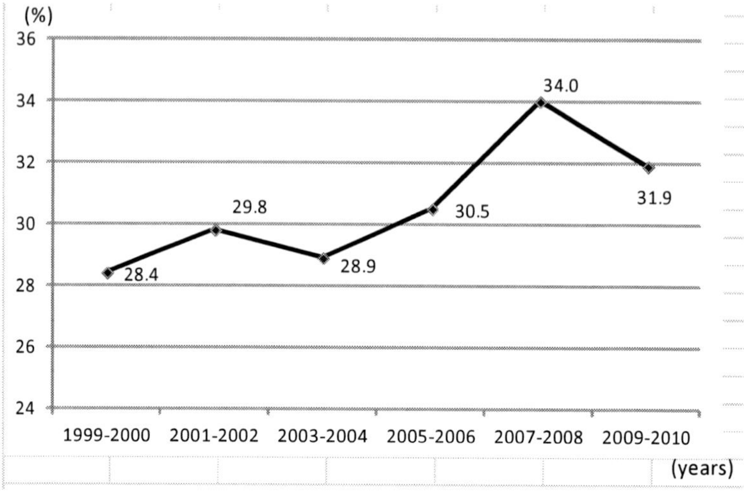

Source: Reference [13].

Figure 1. Prevalence of obesity (BMI $\geq$30 kg/m^2) among U.S. women aged 20-39 y.

The highest prevalence of underweight is reported in underdeveloped regions, such as South Asian or Africa, where undernutrition is generally high owing to food poverty under socio-economic deprivation [20]. High prevalence rates of underweight women are also observed in developed countries such as Japan.

Over the last two decades, the prevalence of underweight Japanese women has increased from 19.6% to 21.2% in those aged 20-29 years, and from 8.6% to 13.3% in those aged 30-39 [21]. A low BMI in women from highly industrialized countries cannot be considered to be a result of environmental factors such as periodic food shortages and malnutrition, but as an expression of constitutional low weight or a result of cosmetically-induced starvation.

Those women often become dissatisfied with their bodies because they are unable to meet the *sociocultural ideal of female beauty*, which prescribes an extremely thin body figure for women. Extreme thinness has been glamorized among reproductive-age women, and unhealthy dieting to lose weight has become a popular practice among them. Body image in younger women is susceptible to societal influence through mass media, such as television, movies, and magazines [22].

Low pre-pregnancy BMI has been associated with a higher incidence of miscarriage [23], delivery of smaller infants [24, 25], and intrauterine growth restriction (IUGR) [2].

Table 1. Obstetrics complications in women with underweight and overweight/obese in pregnant women

	BMI categories (kg/m^2)	
	underweight (<18.5)	overweight (≥25.0) / obesity (≥30.0)
Early pregnancy	Preterm birth	Spontaneous abortion
	Still birth	Congenital anomalies
	miscarriage	miscarriage
Late pregnancy	Preterm delivery	Gesttationa hypertension
	Premature rupture of membranes	Preeclampsia
		Gestational diabetes mellitus
		Preterm delivery
Peripartum		Cesarean delivery
		Failed vaginal bith after cesarean delivery
		Operative morbidities
		Anesthesia complications
		Postpartum endometritis
		Wound breakdown
		Postpartum thrombophlebitis
Fetus, neonate, and offspring	SGA	LGA or Macrosomia
	Low birth weight	Childhood obesity
	Intrauterin growth restriction	Type 2 diabetes
	High neonatal mortality	Metabolic syndrome

SGA, small for gestational age: LGA, large for gestational age

Our previous research among 3,071 Japanese women who gave birth to single-term infants found that underweight women were 1.7 times and 1.5 times more likely to give birth to a small for gestational age (SGA) or low birth weight (LBW) infant, respectively [26]. Furthermore, a study in London found that a BMI of less than 20 kg/m^2 was associated with increased risk of anemia, premature delivery, and LBW [27]. Ehrenberg et al. [2] also observed an increased risk of maternal fever, mediolateral episiotomy, and arrest of active labor among US women with a BMI of less than 19.8 kg/m^2.

RECOMMENDATIONS OF OPTIMAL WEIGHT GAIN DURING PREGNANCY

Adequate weight gain by pre-pregnancy BMI is important for optimal pregnancy outcomes. In 2009, IOM released new recommendations regarding weight gain during pregnancy, as many key aspects of the health of women of childbearing age have changed since the establishment of previous recommendations [28]. These changes include increasingly high rates of overweight and obesity, GWG, and women who become pregnant at an older age. These trends contribute to the risks of poor maternal and child health outcomes.

As a result, women are more commonly entering pregnancy with chronic conditions such as hypertension or diabetes, which put them at risk for pregnancy complications and may lead to increased morbidity during their post-pregnancy years [11].

Compared with previous IOM guidelines, the 2009 IOM recommendations provide upper-weight limits for obese women, and use common adult BMI cutoffs for classifications of weight status. According to the 2009 IOM recommendations, underweight women (BMI<18.5) should gain 12.5-18.0 kg during pregnancy; normal weight women (BMI 18.5-24.9) should gain 11.5-16.0 kg, and overweight women (BMI 25.0-29.9) should gain 7.0-9.0 kg. Nowadays, this is a standard for weight gain worldwide (Table 2) [11]. This new guideline will be used in clinical practice as an effective weight management tool, to help evaluate the association between gestational weight ranges and pregnancy outcomes. Weight gain below the recommended range is associated with low neonatal birth weight, and weight gain above the recommendations is associated with neonatal macrosomia [29]. Appropriate weight gain within the range recommended by the guidelines could improve fetal and maternal outcomes.

Weekly weight gain is also useful for assessing infant growth if mothers do not know their pre-pregnancy body weight or visit antenatal clinics late in the pregnancy. Some studies have reported a strong association between weekly weight gain and the weekly rate of weight gain over a specific trimester. Kruger [30] suggests that pregnant women in developing countries tend to attend antenatal clinics late in pregnancy, so pre-pregnancy BMI may not be known, and antenatal care may have to be provided according to the information of their pregnancy weight gain.

The IOM's new recommendations [11] are based on scientific evidence, and therefore do not include specific recommendations for some women where evidence is lacking, i.e. minority groups, adolescents, and women of short stature.

Further research should be conducted to assess the validity of the new IOM recommendations that are suitable for achieving optimal pregnancy outcomes among both mothers and children.

Table 2. IOM's New Recommendations for total and rate of weight gain during pregnancy by pre-pregnancy BMI

	Total Weight Gain		Rates of Weight Gains* 2nd and 3rd Trimester	
Prepregnancy BMI (kg/m^2)	Range in kg	Range in lbs	Mean (range) in kg/week	Mean (range) in lbs/week
Underweight	12.5-18	28-40	0.51	1
(<18.5)			(0.44-0.58)	(1-1.3)
Normal weight	11.5-16	25-35	0.42	1
(18.5-24.9)			(0.35-0.5)	(0.8-1)
Overweight	7-11.5	15-25	0.28	0..6
(25.0-29.9)			(0.23-0.33)	(0.5-0.7)
Obese	5-9	11-20	0.22	0.5
(≥30.0)			(0.17-0.27)	(0.4-0.6)

* Calculations assume a 0.5-2 kg (1.1-4.4 lbs) weight gain in the first trimester

IOM. Institute of Medicine

MANAGEMENT FOR OBESE WOMEN DURING PREGNANCY

Complications of Obesity during Pregnancy

Obesity is a risk factor for a number of pregnancy complications. There are both short-term and long-term complications for mothers, fetuses, newborns, and for future mothers and children.

(1) Short-term complications

Table 1 summarizes past reports of the perinatal complications of obese pregnant women. Numerous reports [31-35] find an increase in gestational diabetes mellitus (GDM), pregnancy-induced hypertension, macrosomia, surgical delivery, and cesarean section in obese pregnant women, establishing obesity in pregnancy as a high-risk problem. In addiction, there is an increased risk of early miscarriage [14]. Within a diet controlled group, the pre-pregnancy obese group was more likely to have pregnancy-related hypertension (OR=1.56, 95%CI=1.37-1.78) and hyperbilirubinemia (OR=1.29, 95%CI=1.04-1.60) than the non-obese group [36]. Results from a retrospective studies also suggested that obese women have a higher likelihood of postpartum hemorrhage following caesarean (OR=1.73, 95%CI=1.31-2.28) and vaginal (OR=2.11, 95%CI=1.54-2.89) delivery [37].

Other studies also reported the health outcomes of abnormal maternal weight status in special subgroups, such as twin pregnancies and special conditions during pregnancy. For instance, having an obese weight status during pre-pregnancy may be protective against placental abruption for twins pregnancy with OR=0.58, (95% CI=0.38-0.87) when comparing with normal weight US mothers [38]. Pre-pregnancy BMI was associated with LGA with OR=1.25 (95% CI=1.05-1.49) in 86 Canadian Caucasian women with mild glucose intolerance during pregnancy but not gestational diabetes mellitus [39] (116). Nevertheless, a retrospective study in US suggested that maternal obesity is related to a higher chance of cesarean delivery with OR of 2.4 (95%CI=1.9-3.1) [40]. Within pre-pregnancy obese women, the obstructive sleep apnea (OSA) subgroup would have a higher odds of higher infant birth ratio than those without OSA (1.099 vs 1.035) [41].

Furthermore, a recent study has shown that maternal obesity during pregnancy poses a significant risk for the next generation, with metabolic compromise already evident at birth [42]. Newborns born to obese women had a greater percent of body fat, a homeostasis model assessment of insulin resistance, cord leptin, and interleukin-6, when compared to newborns born to lean women. Furthermore, fetal adiposity and insulin resistance had a strong positive correlation, even after adjustment for potential confounders, as were maternal pre-pregnancy BMI and fetal insulin resistance. Cord leptin also correlated significantly with fetal insulin resistance. The overall results of this study have demonstrated that maternal obesity is involved in fetal metabolism.

(2) Long-term complications

There are many reports linking birth weight to increased obesity in adolescents and adults [43, 44]. The Nurse's Health Study [45] reported a slightly greater BMI among adolescent and adult subjects born small, but a much greater prevalence of overweight and obesity in those born large. Subsequently, an increased prevalence of adolescent obesity is well known to be associated with an increased risk of metabolic syndrome. Furthermore, obese women have a high risk for GDM, providing a future risk for type 2 diabetes mellitus.

A systematic review suggested that high GWG could lead to large for gestational age (LGA) and inadequate GWG could lead to SGA [46]. Among >680,000 mother with singleton live births, pre-pregnancy underweight (BMI<18.5) mothers had a higher risk of giving low birth weight (OR = 1.82, 95% CI = 1.77-1.88), very low birth weight (OR = 1.41, 95% CI = 1.31-1.51), SGA (OR = 1.80, 95% CI = 1.76-1.84), preterm (OR = 1.37, 95% CI = 1.33-1.40) and very preterm (OR = 1.42, 95% CI = 1.34-1.50), than non-underweight mothers [47]. Furthermore, pre-pregnancy maternal obesity is related to inflammation problems such as asphyxia in newborns, *as well as respiratory problems in their later childhoods*.

A cross-sectional study in US found that a pre-pregnancy obese status (based on self-reported BMI) is related to having detectable high sensitivity C-reactive protein in children (OR=16.23, 95%CI=2.14-123.12). In a US case-control study, pre-pregnancy weight status was associated with increased risk of childhood respiratory hospitalization, with an adjusted odds ratio OR (95% CI = 1.08 (1.03-1.14) for overweight and OR=1.29 (1.22-1.36) for obese mothers [48]. Consistent findings were reported by longitudinal studies, with the inclusion of GWG and LGA for analyses. According to a 13-year study among 292,568 pre-pregnancy Chinese women, maternal overweight (25.0-29.9 kg/m2) and low gestation weight gain are associated with a slightly higher chance of newborn asphyxia with OR (95%CI) of 1.2 (1.0-1.3) and 1.1 (1.10-1.1), respectively [49].

In another US longitudinal study, LGA and maternal obesity increased the risk of metabolic syndromes including obesity, hypertension, dyslipidemia, and glucose intolerance) with hazard ratios of 2.19 (95% CI: 1.25-3.82) and 1.81 (95% CI: 1.03-3.19), when comparing with appropriate-for-gestational age (AGA) and normal weight status, respectively [50]. When both pre-pregnancy BMI and GWG were considered, a study with 60,892 mothers in Denmark, a high pre-pregnancy BMI and self-reported GWG increased the risk of LGA, but lowered the risk of growth restriction [51]. In another US study among 11,203 mothers, SGA, inadequate GWG was associated with increased odds of SGA (OR=2.51, 95% CI= 1.31-4.78 for underweight and OR 1.78, 95% CI=1.42-2.24 for normal weight women) and decreased odds of LGA (OR 0.5, 95% CI=0.47-0.73 for normal weight and OR=0.56, 95%

CI=0.34-0.90 for obese women). In the same study, excessive GWG was associated with decreased odds of SGA (OR=0.59, 95% CI =0.47-0.73 for normal weight and OR=0.64, 95% CI=0.47-0.89 for overweight women) and increased odds of LGA (OR=1.76, 95% CI=1.38-2.24 for normal weight, OR=2.99, 95% CI=1.92-4.65 for overweight, and OR=1.55, 95% CI=1.10-2.19 for obese women) [52].

PRECAUTIONS IN THE MANAGEMENT OF OBESE PREGNANT WOMEN

(1) Management before pregnancy

As obesity per se is a risk factor for a number of pregnancy complications, obese women should be encouraged to decrease weight before pregnancy. In fact, the American College of Obstetricians and Gynecologists (ACOG) offers their members practical guidelines on how to assess and manage obesity in pregravid women [53]. In the management of obese women before pregnancy, weight loss prior to becoming pregnant through lifestyle improvements, particularly through individualized dietary therapy, appears to be a useful approach. Counseling to support improvements in diet and physical activity is considered to be a first-line intervention. The U.S. Preventive Services Task Force found that the most successful nonsurgical approaches were intensive, weight-focused counseling and multicomponent, intensive interventions that combined nutrition and exercise counseling [54]. The implementation of this approach, however, must be confirmed by a randomized control trial, which is not available up to date.

(2) Management during pregnancy

The recommendations for weight gain during pregnancy have been based on the IOM guidelines published in 2009 [11]. These guidelines were initially established to help decrease the risk of fetal growth restriction. On the other hand, there are no evidence-based nutritional guidelines for obese women in pregnancy. There have been conflicting ideas in the past about whether or not to restrict energy intake for obese pregnant women. The current line of thought is not to restrict energy intake in the extreme condition because there is no evidence about how this might affect the long-term outcome for the infant. In particular, dietary restrictions that lead to positive ketones in urine should be avoided. This is because of the possibility that a high ketone concentration may negatively affect the infant's intelligence [55]. The ACOG recommends that nutrition consultation be offered to all obese women, and that they should be encouraged to follow an exercise program. This consultation should continue postpartum and before attempting another pregnancy [56].

Various perinatal complications are known to develop more frequently in obese pregnant women, and it is particularly important to screen for and prevent from maternal, delivery, and neonatal complications. Lifestyle improvement before pregnancy is essential, but an appropriate level of energy intake without extra weight gains appears to be a valid individual adaptation to pregnancy management. GDM, a clinical manifestation of glucose intolerance in pregnancy, is associated with perinatal complication The pathophysiology of GDM involves both decreased insulin sensitivity and insufficiency of insulin secretion, resulting in hyperglycemia. Obese women are generally more insulin resistant compared with non-obese women, whether during the pregravid period or pregnancy, and there are significant decreases in maternal insulin sensitivity by the end of the pregnancy [57]. The fact that decreased insulin sensitivity causes the limited ability of insulin to transport glucose from the intravascular into peripheral tissues such as skeletal muscle and adipose, suggests the greater risk of developing GDM in obese women than others.

Therefore, in the management of obese pregnant women, consideration should be given to screening for GDM in the first trimester and repeating it later in pregnancy if the initial screening result is negative. This screening would be helpful for women who have other risk factors for GDM, such as a previous history of GDM, a family history of type 2 diabetes or macrosomia, etc.

The number of obese women of childbearing age considering bariatric surgery is increasing, resulting in questions about pregnancy after these types of surgeries. It has been reported that pregnancy after bariatric surgery is less likely to be complicated by gestational diabetes, hypertension, macrosomia, and cesarean delivery than pregnancy of obese women who did not receive the bariatric surgery [58, 59]. However, women who have undergone bariatric surgery often experience deficiencies in iron, vitamin B12, folate, and calcium. Therefore, consideration should be given to prescribing supplementation of vitamin B12, folate, iron, and calcium to women who have undergone bariatric surgery.

Nevertheless, up-to-date information may suggest that maintaining a healthy weight status before and during pregnancy is critical to mothers' and children health. There are several ways of maintaining a healthy weight status in women before pregnancy. Obesity screening programs for reproductive-aged women should be advocated [60]. For smokers and alcohol drinkers, improvement of nutrition and exercise through cessation programs could be an effective way of maintaining a normal pre-pregnancy body weight status [61].

Low Weight Gain during Pregnancy and Perinatal Complications

Under-nutrition and imbalanced diet can contribute to low gestational weight gain. Low weight gain not only leads to adverse health outcomes in mothers and infants, but also in women with low pre-pregnancy BMI. These adverse outcomes were observed in most studies, which reports that low gestational weight gain is associated with an increased risk of SGA infants and prenatal mortality [29, 62]. Low pre-pregnancy BMI is also associated with a higher incidence of miscarriage [23] and the delivery of smaller infants [24, 25].

There is strong evidence for the association between weight gains below the recommended level of IOM guidelines and the risk of having an SGA infant [63, 64]. In a study among 26,028 women in California, those with gestational weight gains below that recommended by the IOM guidelines had a significantly higher risk of SGA infants when compared with women with weight gains above the recommended level, after adjusting for pre-pregnancy BMI. GWG of less than 7 kg was also associated with increased risk of infantile seizure, hospital stay of more than five days, and SGA [65]. Furthermore, longitudinal findings are available from a population-based retrospective cohort study among 570,672 U.S. women aged 18-40 years, examining the association between the 2009 IOM recommendations and adverse infant outcomes by pre-pregnancy BMI [64]. Twenty-two percent of women were below the recommended weight gain by the IOM guidelines, and the proportion of SGA decreased with increased weight gain during pregnancy for all BMI groups.

In addition, gains of less than the recommended level were associated with increased odds of SGA (adjusted OR range: 1.11-2.97), and gains greater than the recommended level were associated with decreased odds of SGA (adjusted

OR range: 0.38-0.83). In a study among 3,870 pregnant US women, Caulfield et al. [66] found that women with weight gains lower than the IOM recommended ranges, are more likely to be black, young, short, thin, and less educated smokers. In another study in North Carolina, Mumford et al. [67] found an association between restricted eating and weight gain during pregnancy. Women with BMIs of more than 19.8 kg/m^2 and a history of dieting or restricted eating gained more weight during pregnancy. In contrast, underweight women with a history of restricted eating behaviors gained less weight compared to underweight women without those behaviors.

In non-US populations, similar results were also observed. In Sweden, women with a singleton full-term birth have higher risks of SGA when gaining <8 kg (adjusted OR range: 1.68-2.35) and lower risks of SGA when gaining >16 kg (adjusted OR range: 0.50-0.61) [65]. In Asia, Merchant et al. [68] also reported lower mean birth weight of newborns among Pakistani women with pre-pregnancy BMI<19 kg/m^2 who gained>12.5 kg compared to those who gained 12.5 kg. Indian women in the lowest quartile for both pre-pregnancy BMI and GWG were 5.6 times more likely to have IUGR infants, compared to the upper quartile [69]. Therefore, a positive association may exist between infant birth weight and GWG which decreased with higher pre-pregnancy BMI.

The above evidence indicates that gestational weight gain, particularly during the second and third trimesters, is an important determinant of fetal growth [70, 71]. Inadequate weight gains during these trimesters are associated with an increased risk of LBW or IUGR. Health care providers should provide women individual records of their weight gains at each antenatal check-up, as a valuable source of dietary information.

Short-and Long-term Effects of Fetal Environment for Offspring

Many animal models have demonstrated that altering the environment in utero can have lifelong consequences, such as adiposity, fat distribution, sarcopenia, insulin sensitivity, glucose intolerance, and high blood pressure (BP) [7, 8, 30, 72]. Population-based prospective cohort studies tracking from the preconceptional or early fetal stages to young adulthood seem to be a more suitable epidemiological design (Figure 2) [73, 74]. A UK prospective pregnancy cohort study in 5,154 mother-offspring pairs examined the associations of GWG and pre-pregnancy weight with offspring adiposity and cardiovascular risk factors. Women who gained more weight than recommended by the 2009 IOM GWG had offspring of higher adiposity, systolic blood pressure, C-reactive protein, and IL-6, and of lower HDL-C and apolipoprotein A1 levels at the age of nine years old [7]. An Australia population-based birth cohort study in 2,432 mother-offspring pairs examined the associations between maternal GWG and offspring BMI and BP at 21 years of age. Offspring BMI was on average 0.3 kg/m^2 higher for each 0.1 kg/w GWG greater than the 2009 IOM recommended GWG values, after adjustment for potential confounding factors.

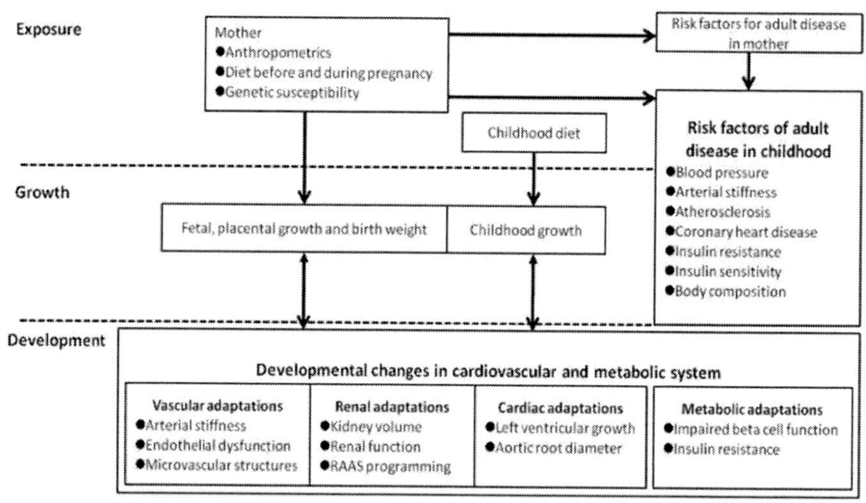

Sources; References [73, 74].

Figure 2. Models for studying the fetal origins of adult diseases hypotheses in epidemiological studies. This models presents the core associations factors that have to be studied to unravel the underlying mechanisms of the associations between fetal growth restriction and low birth weight, and disease in later life. RAAS, Renin-angiotensin-aldosterone system.

Systolic BP was also greater (0.2 mmHg pre 0.1 kg) in offspring whose mothers had higher GWG. As a summary, greater GWG was associated with greater offspring BMI and higher systolic BP in offspring [8].

Studies in humans generally use birth weight as a measure of adverse fetal exposure. Birth weight might indeed be an indicator of the quality of the intrauterine environment [75]. A number of mechanistic frameworks have been proposed to explain the biological basis of the possible associations observed between low birth weight and obesity in later life in epidemiological, clinical and experimental animal studies [76]. Hales et al. [77] coined the "*thrifty phenotype*" hypothesis, which suggested that when the fetal environment is undernourished. There is an adaptive response, which optimizes the size of body growth in utero and leads to a permanently altered postnatal metabolism, which is designed to enhance postnatal survival under conditions of intermittent or long-lasting poor nutrient supply.

Systematic reviews show that indicators of low GWG caused by nutritional deficit in pregnancy are associated with greater risk of diabetes and cardiovascular mortality. In one recent systematic review, infants who are born small, show rapid catch-up growth and become obese in later life [78]. Stettler et al. suggested that catch-up growth in the first few weeks of postnatal life is particularly disadvantageous for adult obesity [79, 80]. Another systematic review relating to the birth weight/type 2 diabetes relationship noted that for every one-kg increase in weight at birth, the risk of diabetes in adulthood decreased by 25% (OR=0.75, 95% CI=0.70-0.81) [81].

In a study among Indian young adults, which followed up subjects every six months from birth to, until the age of 21 years, shown that plasma glucose concentrations and insulin resistance were inversely related to birthweight, and impaired glucose tolerance and diabetes were associated with lower weight and BMI at the age of 1 year, after adjusting for adult BMI [82]. The findings from these available studies suggested that minor perturbation of inadequate maternal nutritional status can program fetal development. This programming is a product of altered expression of key genes, possibly driving the tissue remodeling response and future disease risk.

There are limitations to generalize the available findings on the associations of pregnancy weight status and health outcomes in mothers and children to clinical practices. First, such associations may vary across different geographic areas, i.e. different socioeconomic factors exist. Moreover, BMI was used as the sole anthropometric indicator of weight status, important central obesity indicators such as waist circumference [83] was seldom used. In some studies, self-reported BMI values were used. It is also not clear which pre-pregnancy weight status (underweight, normal weight, or overweight) actually has a relatively higher GWG, although the obese group seems to have the least GWG [84]. Furthermore, the independent and synergic effects of pre-pregnancy weight status and GWG on the health of mothers and their next generations (infants and childhood) are even complex. In some cases, the overall program will be complicated by the existence of maternal insulin resistance and gestational diabetes. More well-designed longitudinal studies are certainly warranted.

Conclusion

Pre-pregnancy BMI and pregnancy weigh gain reflect maternal nutritional status before and during pregnancy, which plays a crucial role in creating an optimal intrauterine environment. Understanding the relationship between maternal nutrition and birth outcomes may provide a foundation for developing nutritional interventions that will improve birth outcomes and long-term quality of life. The fetal origins hypothesis proposes that inadequate maternal nutrition and low infant birth weight can predispose the child to diseases such as diabetes and cardiovascular disease later in life. Pregnancy can be a good time to improve one's nutrition and participate in health activities. All women of reproductive age are encouraged to follow the dietary recommendations and maintain a well-balanced diet. To improve birth outcomes, it is critical for women to modify their health behaviors for a better nutritional status before, during, and after conception.

References

[1] Neggers Y, Goldenberg RL. Some thoughts on body mass index, micronutrient intakes and pregnancy outcome. *J. Nutr.,* 2003; 133: 1737S-40S.

[2] Ehrenberg HM, Dierker L, Milluzzi C, Mercer BM. Low maternal weight, failure to thrive in pregnancy, and adverse pregnancy outcomes. *Am. J. Obstet. Gynecol.,* 2003; 189: 1726-30.

[3] Margerison Zilko CE, Rehkopf D, Abrams B. Association of maternal gestational weight gain with short-and long-term maternal and child health outcomes. *Am. J. Obstet. Gynecol.,* 2010; 202: 574.e1-8.

[4] Oken E, Kleinman KP, Belfort MB, Hammitt JK, Gillman MW. Associations of gestational weight gain with short-and longer-term maternal and child health outcomes. *Am. J. Epidemiol.,* 2009; 170: 173-80.

[5] Saldana TM, Siega-Riz AM, Adair LS. Effect of macronutrient intake on the development of glucose intolerance during pregnancy. *Am. J. Clin. Nutr.,* 2004; 79: 479-86.

[6] Goldfrey KM, Barker DJ. Fetal nutrition and adult disease. *Am. J. Clin. Nutr.,* 2000; 71: 1344S-52S.

[7] Fraser A, Tilling K, Macdonald-Wallis C, et al. Association of maternal weight gain in pregnancy with offspring obesity and metabolic and vascular traits in childhood. *Circulation,* 2010; 121: 2557-64.

[8] Mamun AA, O'Callaghan M, Callaway L, et al. Associations of gestational weight gain with offspring body mass index and blood pressure at 21 years of age: evidence from a birth cohort study. *Circulation,* 2009; 119: 1720-7.

[9] Laraia BA, Bodnar LM, Siega-Riz AM. Pregaravid body mass index is negatively associated with diet quality during pregnancy. *Public Health Nutr.,* 2007; 10: 920-6.

[10] Olafsdottir AS, Skuladottir GV, Thorsdottir I, et al. Maternal diet in early and late pregnancy in relation to weight gain. *Int. J. Obes.,* 30; 2006: 492-9.

[11] Institute of Medicine. Weight gain during pregnancy: reexamining the guidelines, Washington, DC: National Academies Press; 2009.

[12] World Health Organization. Obesity: preventing and managing a global epidemic. *World Health Organ Tech. Rep. Ser.,* 2000; 894:1–4.

[13] Flegal KM, Carroll MD, Kit BK, Ogden CL. Prevalence of obesity and trends in the distribution of body mass index among US adults, 1999-2010. *JAMA,* 2012; 307: 491-7.

[14] Lashen H, Fear K, Sturdee DW. Obesity is associated with increased risk of first trimester and recurrent miscarriage: matched case-control study. *Hum. Reprod.,* 2004; 19: 1644-6.

[15] Van der Steeg JW, Steures P, Eijkemans MJ, et al. Obesity affects spontaneous pregnancy chances in subfertile, ovulatory women. *Hum. Reprod.,* 2008; 23: 324-8.

[16] Usha Kiran TS, Hemmadi S, Bethel J, Evans J. Outcome of pregnancy in a women with an increased body mass index. BJOG 2005; 112: 768-72.

[17] Andreasen KR, Andersen ML, Schantz AL. Obesity and pregnancy. *Acta. Obstet. Gynecol. Scand.,* 2004; 83: 1022-9.

[18] Heslehurst N, Ells LJ, Simpson H, Batterham A, Wilkinson J, Summerbell CD. Trends in maternal obesity incidence rates, demographic predictors, and health inequalities in 36,821 women over a 15-year period. *BJOG,* 2007; 114: 187-94.

[19] Australian Institute of Health and Welfare (AIHW). Australia's health 2010: The eighth biannual health report of the AIHW. Australian Institute of Health and Welfare, Canberra; 2010.

[20] Macro International Inc. Measure DHS, Demographic and Health Surveys; 2007. http://www.measuredhs.com/countries/ [Accessed December 1, 2010].

[21] Hayashi F, Takimoto H, Yoshita K, Yoshiike N. Perceived body size and desire for thinness of young Japanese women: a population-based survey. *Br. J. Nutr.,* 2006; 96: 1154-62.

[22] Wadsworth LA, Johnson CP. Mass media and healthy aging. *J. Nutr. Elder.,* 2008; 27: 319-31.

[23] Helgstrand S, Andersen AM. Maternal underweight and the risk of spontaneous abortion. *Acta. Obstet. Gynecol. Scand.,* 2005; 84, 1197-201.

[24] Sekiya N, Anai T, Matsubara M, Miyazaki F. Maternal weight gain rate in the second trimester are associated with birth weight and length of gestation. *Gynecol. Obstet. Invest.,* 2007; 63: 45-8.

[25] Watanabe H, Inoue K, Doi M, et al. Risk factors for term small for gestational age infants in women with low pre-pregnancy body mass index. *J. Obstet. Gynecol. Res.,* 2010; 36: 506-12.

[26] Watanabe H, Fukuoka H, Inoue K, et al. Restricting weight gain during pregnancy in Japan: a controversial factor in reducing perinatal complications. *Eur. J. Obstet. Gynecol. Reprod. Biol.,* 2007; 133: 53-9.

[27] Sebire NJ, Jolly M, Harris JP, Regan L, Robinson S. Is maternal underweight really a risk factor for adverse pregnancy outcome? A population-based study in London. *BJOG,* 2001; 108: 61-6.

[28] Institute of Medicine. Nutrition during pregnancy. Washington, DC: National Academies Press; 1990: 10-23.

[29] Parker JD, Abrams B. Prenatal weight gain advice: an examination of the recent prenatal weight gain recommendations of the Institute of Medicine. *Obstet. Gynecol.,* 1992; 79: 664-9.

[30] Kruger HS. Maternal anthropometry and pregnancy outcomes: a proposal for the monitoring of pregnancy weight gain in outpatient clinics in South Africa. *Curationis,* 2005; 28: 40-9.

[31] Castro LC, Avina RL. Maternal obesity and pregnancy outcomes. *Curr. Opin. Obstet. Gynecol.,* 2002; 14: 601-6.

[32] Wall PD, Deucy EE, Glantz JC, Pressman EK. Vertical skin incisions and wound complications in the obese parturient. *Obstet. Gynecol.,* 2003; 102: 952-6.

[33] Rosenberg TJ, Garbers S, Chavkin W, Chiasson MA. Pre-pregnancy weight and adverse perinatal outcomes in an ethnically diverse population. *Obstet. Gynecol.,* 2003; 102: 1022-7.

[34] Jensen DM, Damm P, Sorensen B, et al. Pregnancy outcome and pre-pregnancy body mass index in 2459 glucose-tolerant Danish women. *Am. J. Obstet. Gynecol.,* 2003; 189: 239-44.

[35] O'Brien TE, Ray JG, Chan WS. Maternal body mass index and the risk of preeclampsia: a systemic overview. *Epidemiology,* 2003; 14: 368-74.

[36] Joy S, Roman A, Istwan N, Rhea D, Desch C, Stanziano G, et al. The effect of maternal obesity on pregnancy outcomes of women with gestational diabetes controlled with diet only, glyburide, or insulin. *Am. J. Perinatol.,* 2012; 29(8): 643-8.

[37] Fyfe EM, Thompson JM, Anderson NH, Groom KM, McCowan LM. Maternal obesity and postpartum haemorrhage after vaginal and caesarean delivery among nulliparous women at term: a retrospective cohort study. *BMC Pregnancy Childbirth,* 2012; 12(1):112.

[38] Aliyu MH, Alio AP, Lynch O, Mbah A, Salihu HM. Maternal pre-gravid body weight and risk for placental abruption among twin pregnancies. *J. Matern. Fetal. Neonatal. Med.,* 2009; 22(9): 745-50.

[39] Segal P, Hamilton JK, Sermer M, Connelly PW, Hanley AJ, Zinman B, et al. Maternal obesity and familial history of diabetes have opposing effects on infant birth weight in women with mild glucose intolerance in pregnancy. *J. Matern. Fetal. Neonatal. Med.,* 2008; 21(1): 73-9.

[40] Chin JR, Henry E, Holmgren CM, Varner MW, Branch DW. Maternal obesity and contraction strength in the first stage of labor. *Am. J. Obstet. Gynecol.,* 2012; 207(2): 129 e1-6.

[41] Olivarez SA, Ferres M, Antony K, Mattewal A, Maheshwari B, Sangi-Haghpeykar H, et al. Obstructive sleep apnea screening in pregnancy, perinatal outcomes, and impact of maternal obesity. *Am. J. Perinatol.,* 2011; 28(8): 651-8.

[42] Catalano PM, Presley L, Minium J, Hauguel-de Mouzon S. Fetuses of obese mothers develop insulin resistance in utero. *Diabetes Care,* 2009; 32:1076-80.

[43] Garn SM, Clark DC. Trends in fatness and the origins of obesity. *Pediatrics,* 1976; 57: 443–56.

[44] Garn SM, Cole PE, Bailey SM. Living together as a factor in family line resemblances. *Hum. Biol.,* 1979; 51: 565–87.

[45] Curhan GC, Chertow GM, Willett WC, et al. Birth weight and adult hypertension and obesity in women. *Circulation,* 1996; 94: 1310–5.

[46] Siega-Riz AM, Viswanathan M, Moos MK, Deierlein A, Mumford S, Knaack J, et al. A systematic review of outcomes of maternal weight gain according to the Institute of Medicine recommendations: birthweight, fetal growth, and postpartum weight retention. *Am. J. Obstet. Gynecol.,* 2009; 201(4): 339 e1-14.

[47] Salihu HM, Lynch O, Alio AP, Mbah AK, Kornosky JL, Marty PJ. Extreme maternal underweight and feto-infant morbidity outcomes: a population-based study. *J. Matern. Fetal. Neonatal. Med.,* 2009; 22(5): 428-34.

[48] Parsons EC, Patel K, Tran BT, Littman AJ. Maternal Pre-Gravid Obesity and Early Childhood Respiratory Hospitalization: A Population-Based Case-Control Study. *Matern. Child Health J.,* 2012 Aug 18 [Epub ahead of print].

[49] Liu Y, Dai W, Dai X, Li Z. Pre-pregnancy body mass index and gestational weight gain with the outcome of pregnancy: a 13-year study of 292,568 cases in China. *Arch. Gynecol. Obstet.,* 2012; 286(4): 905-11.

[50] Boney CM, Verma A, Tucker R, Vohr BR. Metabolic syndrome in childhood: association with birth weight, maternal obesity, and gestational diabetes mellitus. *Pediatrics,* 2005; 115(3): e290-6.

[51] Nohr EA, Vaeth M, Baker JL, Sorensen T, Olsen J, Rasmussen KM. Combined associations of pre-pregnancy body mass index and gestational weight gain with the outcome of pregnancy. *Am. J. Clin. Nutr.,* 2008; 87(6): 1750-9.

[52] Simas TA, Waring ME, Liao X, Garrison A, Sullivan GM, Howard AE, et al. Pre-pregnancy weight, gestational weight gain, and risk of growth affected neonates. *J. Womens Health (Larchmt),* 2012; 21(4): 410-7.

[53] The role of the obstetrician-gynecologist in the assessment and management of obesity. ACOG Committee Opinion No. 319. American College of Obstetricians and Gynecologists. *Obstet. Gynecol.,* 2005; 106: 895–9.

[54] Screening for obesity in adults: recommendations and rationale. U.S. Preventive Services Task Force. *Ann. Intern. Med.,* 2003; 139: 930–2.

[55] Rizzo T, Metzger BE, Burns WJ, Burns K. Correlations between antepartum maternal metabolism and child intelligence. *N. Engl. J. Med.,* 1991; 325: 911-6.

[56] Obesity in pregnancy. ACOG Committee Opinion No. 315. American College of Obstetricians and Gynecologists. *Obstet. Gynecol.,* 2005; 106: 671–5.

[57] Catalano PM, Ehrenberg HM. The short- and long-term implications of maternal obesity on the mother and her offspring. *BJOG,* 2006; 113: 1126–33.

[58] Sheiner E, Levy A, Silverberg D, et al. Pregnancy after bariatric surgery is not associated with adverse perinatal outcome. *Am. J. Obstet. Gynecol.,* 2004; 190: 1335–40.

[59] Martin LF, Finigan KM, Nolan TE. Pregnancy after adjustable gastric banding. *Obstet. Gynecol.,* 2000; 95: 927–30.

[60] Zera C, McGirr S, Oken E. Screening for obesity in reproductive-aged women. *Prev. Chronic. Dis.,* 2011; 8(6): A125.

[61] Emerson MH, Glovsky E, Amaro H, Nieves R. Unhealthy weight gain during treatment for alcohol and drug use in four residential programs for Latina and African American women. *Subst. Use Misuse*, 2009; 44(11): 1553-65.

[62] Taffel SM. Maternal weight gain and the outcome of pregnancy. *Vital. Health Stat.,* 21 1986; 44: 1-25.

[63] Nielsen JN, O'Brien KO, Witter FR, et al. High gestational weight gain does not improve birth weight in a cohort of African American adolescents. *Am. J. Clin. Nutr.,* 2006; 84: 183-9.

[64] Park S, Sappenfield WM, Bish C, Salihu H, Goodman D, Bensyl DM. Assessment of the Institute of Medicine Recommendations for Weight Gain During Pregnancy: Florida, 2004-2007. *Matern. Child Health J.,* 2010 Mar 20 [Epub ahead of print].

[65] Cedergren M. Effects of gestational weight gain and body mass index on obstetrics outcome in Sweden. *Int. J. Gynaecol. Obstet.,* 2006; 93: 269-74.

[66] Caulfield LE, Witter FR, Stoltzfus RJ. Determinants of gestational weight Gain outside the recommended ranges among black and white women. *Obstet. Gynecol.,* 1996; 87: 760-6.

[67] Mumford SL, Siega-Riz AM, Herring A, Evenson KR. Dietary restraint and gestational weight gain. *J. Am. Diet Assoc.,* 2008; 108: 1646-53.

[68] Merchant SS, Momin I A, Sewani AA, Zuberi N F. Effect of pre-pregnancy body mass index and gestational weight gain on birth weight. *J. Pak. Med. Assoc.,* 1999; 49: 23–5.

[69] Naidu AN, Rao NP. Body mass index: a measure of the nutritional status in Indian populations. *Eur. J. Clin. Nutr.,* 1994; 48 (Suppl 3): S131-40.

[70] Kaiser L, Allen LH, American Diabetic Association. Position of the American Dietic Association: nutrition and lifestyle for a healthy pregnancy outcome. *J. Am. Diet Assoc.,* 2008; 108: 553-61.

[71] Althuizen E, van Poppel MN, Seidell JC, van der Wijden, van Mechelen W. Design of the New Life (style) study: a randomized controlled trial to optimize maternal weight development during pregnancy. *BMJ Public Health,* 2006; 6: 168.

[72] Lindsay RS, Nelson SM, Walker JD, et al. Programming of adiposity in offspring of mothers with type 1 diabetes at age 7 years. *Diabetes Care,* 2010; 33: 1080-5.

[73] Jaddoe VW, Witteman JC. Hypotheses on the fetal origins of adult diseases: contributions of epidemiological studies. *Eur. J. Epidemiol.,* 2006; 21: 91-102.

[74] Geelhoed JJ, Jaddoe VW. Early influences on cardiovascular and renal development. *Eur. J. Epidemiol.,* 2010; 25: 677-92.

[75] Brooks AA, Johnson MR, Steer PJ, Pawson ME, Abdalla HI. Birth weigh: nature or nurture ? *Early Hum. Dev.,* 1995; 42: 29-35.

[76] Mühlhäusler BS, Adam CL, McMillen IC. Maternal nutrition and the programming of obesity: *The brain. Organogenesis,* 2008; 4: 144-52.

[77] Hales CN, Barker DJ. The thrifty phenotype hypothesis. *Br. Med. Bull.,* 2001; 60: 5-20.

[78] Ong KK, Loos RJ. Rapid infancy weight gain and subsequent obesity: systematic reviews and hopeful suggestions. *Acta. Paediatr.,* 2006; 95: 904-8.

[79] Stettler N, Kumanyika SK, Katz SH, Zemel BS, Stallings VA. Rapid weight gain during infancy and obesity in young adulthood in a cohort of African Americans. *Am. J. Clin. Nutr.,* 2003; 77: 1374-8.

[80] Stettler N, Stallings VA, Troxel AB, et al. Weight gain in the first week of life and overweight in adulthood: a cohort study of European American subjects fed infant formula. *Circulation,* 2005; 111: 1897-903.

[81] Whincup PH, Kaye SJ, Owen CG, et al. Birth weight and risk of type 2 diabetes: a systematic review. *JAMA,* 2008; 300: 2886-97.

[82] Bhargava SK, Sachdev HS, Fall CH, et al. Relation of serial changes in childhood body mass index to impaired glucose tolerance in young adulthood. *N. Eng. J. Med.,* 2004; 350: 865-75.

[83] Kumar S, Han J, Li T, Qureshi AA. Obesity, waist circumference, weight change and the risk of psoriasis in US women. *J. Eur. Acad. Dermatol. Venereol.,* 2012; Oct 12 [Epub ahead of print].

[84] Chu SY, Callaghan WM, Bish CL, D'Angelo D. Gestational weight gain by body mass index among US women delivering live births, 2004-2005: fueling future obesity. *Am. J. Obstet. Gynecol.,* 2009; 200(3): 271 e1-7.

In: Weight Gain
Editors: A. Pirotte and T. Libert
ISBN: 978-1-62618-800-6

Chapter 3

WOMEN'S PERCEPTIONS OF POSTPARTUM WEIGHT RETENTION AND THEIR BODY IMAGE IN RELATION TO BREASTFEEDING OUTCOMES IN JAPAN

Madoka Inoue and Colin W. Binns
Curtin University, Perth, Western Australia, Australia

ABSTRACT

Weight retention in the postpartum period is a concern for many women following the increase in weight during pregnancy and they often struggle to return to pre-pregnancy levels. Postpartum weight retention may lead to obesity that is then associated with increased rates of several chronic diseases, including type 2 diabetes and cardiovascular disease. Prolonged breastfeeding is believed to help with weight loss during the postpartum period. Breastfeeding and in particular, 'exclusive breastfeeding' for the first six month of life, provides a wide range of health benefits for infants but also to mothers. Most pediatric organizations recommend exclusive breastfeeding for six months and then continuing for as long as the mother desires.

In Japan, women's body image has a strong influence on control of their weight due to the prevailing cultural norm that 'being slim is beautiful'. This is an important factor when considering postpartum weight retention together with breastfeeding practices. Japan has the least number of women who are overweight among all of the developed countries. But despite this many Japanese women perceive themselves to be overweight, both before and after pregnancy. While they of necessity increase their weight during pregnancy, many undertake activities to regain pre-pregnancy body shape soon after birth due to their desire to regain their ideal body image of being slim. A study of Japanese postpartum women residing in Himeji-city, (n = 1,612) showed that more than 42% of women believed that they had not yet returned to their weight at 18 months postpartum, even though 18% were actually in the 'underweight range (Body Mass Index $\leq$ 18.5)'. The women who had returned to their pre-pregnancy weight stated that their weight loss usually occurred within six months after birth (59.6%), during the time when most were breastfeeding. In the study, the postpartum women were asked about their level of concern about body appearance using the Attention to Body Shape Scale (ABS). The average score of the ABS was 24.2 (Standard Deviation [SD] = 4.2) suggesting that postpartum women in Japan were highly conscious about their body shape. Women' body image is related to infant feeding practices as breastfeeding is associated with weight loss, but also breastfeeding may be associated with breast shape changes and hence changes in body image. In this chapter, we describe and discuss women's perceptions of postpartum weight retention and their body image in relation to breastfeeding outcomes, particularly focusing on a trend in Japan.

Keywords: Weight retention, postpartum women, breastfeeding, body image, Japan

1. Introduction

Postpartum weight retention is a concern for many women as they often struggle to return their pre-pregnancy weight after the birth of their child (Montgomery et al., 2011). Postpartum weight retention is a predictor of being overweight or obese in the future and this may be associated with several health problems including metabolic syndrome, hyperlipidemia, and hypertension (Lee et al., 2001). These are well established risk factors for non-communicable diseases including type 2 diabetes, cardiovascular disease and cancer. Postpartum weight retention may also affect women's mental health. Obese or overweight women are more likely to develop postpartum depression (Herring et al., 2008). It has also been reported that prolonged breastfeeding, particularly 'exclusive breastfeeding', that is feeding breastmilk only to infants, with no other liquids, for at least six months helps with a weight reduction of women during the postpartum period (Baker et al., 2008; Kac, Benicio, Velasquez-Melendez, Valente, & Struchiner, 2004). However, in many countries average breastfeeding duration is shorter than the period recommended by the World Health Organization (WHO).

In Japan, the 2010 National Survey of Infants' Growth, which has been carried out every decade since 1960, has reported that more than 55% of mothers continued 'exclusive breastfeeding' at four-five months (Minister of Health Labour and Walfare, 2011). However, as the standard WHO definitions of breastfeeding were not used in the National Surveys, it is difficult to interpret this result. Japan is known to have least number of women who are overweight or obese in the Western Pacific region. In 2011, the World Health Organization (WHO) reported that the prevalence of obesity or overweight (Body Mass Index [BMI] $\geq$ 25 kg/m^2) in women during 2002-2010 for countries in the Western Pacific Region. Japan had the lowest reported rates (See Table 1).

While almost all countries in this region have had increases in the prevalence of overweight or obesity in women over the last eight years, only Japan has shown a reverse trend, with a decrease in the proportion of the overweight or obese population (See Table 1). Several researchers have argued that the trend for increasing weight in Asia is linked to an increase in westernized diets that are high fat, high sugar and low fiber, together with a decrease in physical activity (Drewnowski, 2000; Popkin, 2004). In a study reviewing changes in the BMI of Japanese women over the last 60 years, Sugawara et al (2009) analyzed the "Japanese trend", a decrease of women's BMI since the 1970s, a period during which Japan has had rapid economic growth, lifestyle changes, and increased media exposure to the western cultures. In recent decades, many other Asian countries have also improved their economic and nutritional status but they have not experienced the same trend as Japan for women's body weight and BMI.

When considering postpartum weight retention and breastfeeding outcomes in Japan, psychological and cultural factors, including women's body image, need to be taken into account because of their influence on the control of body weight (Yoshiike, Kaneda, & Takimoto, 2002). The cultural belief in Japan, "being slim is beautiful" places pressure on Japanese women to maintain their weight regardless of age and birth experiences. In a review of postpartum weight retention among Asian women (excluding Japan), Cheng et al (2011) recommended that studies be undertaken on postpartum weight retention. However, there are few published studies available in the literature on postpartum weight retention in Japan. The aim of this chapter is to review available studies and to describe trends in Japanese women's perceptions of postpartum weight retention and their body image in relation to breastfeeding outcomes.

Table 1. The trend in the prevalence (%) of overweight or obesity (BMI ≥ 25 kg/m²) by age in Asian women during 2002-2010

Country/year	Above 15 years old (> 15) (%)			Above 30 years old (>30) (%)		
	2002	2005	2010	2002	2005	2010
China	22.7	24.7	32.0	28.1	30.1	37.9
South Korea	38.2	43.8	53.8	48.1	51.0	60.7
Singapore	20.7	22.0	26.7	23.9	25.4	30.3
Malaysia	34.2	37.2	42.2	42.5	45.7	50.9
Philippine	25.4	28.5	33.6	30.2	33.5	38.9
Viet Nam	7.0	8.7	12.2	10.5	13.0	18.1
New Zealand	64.0	68.2	74.2	71.2	74.6	79.5
Australia	60.2	62.7	66.5	67.1	69.2	72.5
Japan	18.6	18.1	16.2	25.7	25.2	22.2

Source: (Word Health Organization, 2011).

2. Postpartum Weight Retention and Women's Body Image in Japan

A decrease in the prevalence (%) of overweight and obesity in Japan does not indicate an increase in the proportion of women with 'normal' BMI in women, but reflects a shift to the left of the BMI distribution curve, resulting in an increase in the proportion classified as having an 'underweight' BMI. The proportion of Japanese women in the 'underweight' BMI category aged 20-29 and 30-39 years has increased from 12.4% and 7.8% in 1980 to 22.3% and 14.4% in 2009, respectively (Ministry of Health Labour and Walfare, 2002; Ministry of Health Labour and Welfare, 2010). This government study reported that more than half of the women in these age groups overestimated their weight and thought they were obese and thus attempted to reduced their weight inappropriately (Ministry of Health Labour and Welfare, 2009). In a study of 1,731 non- pregnant and non-lactating women aged 15-39 years, Hayashi et al. (2006) found that more than 40% of Japanese women, regardless of their age, desired to be slim and this desire was more common in women aged 35-39 years compared with women aged 25-29 years (Odds Ratio [OR] = 2.74; 95% CI = 1.93-3.89), even though they were within the 'normal' range for BMI. Although, Japanese women have been reported to be relatively conscious about their body weight and shape, there are few published studies on postpartum weight retention in Japan (Hayashi, et al., 2006). In a small recent cross-sectional study of 67 Japanese women investigating postpartum weigh retention at 18-36 months post birth, 13% of women who were in the 'underweight' BMI category before pregnancy remained in the same category at the time of survey, while 4% changed their BMI category from 'normal', pre-pregnancy, to 'underweight' post birth (E. Watanabe, Lee, Kawakubo, & Marui, 2008). In this study, the average weight retention from before their first pregnancy to the survey time (18-36 months postpartum) was1.83 kg (E. Watanabe, et al., 2008). In a large study of Japanese postpartum women aged 30-65 years (n = 1,955), the average weight retention was 1.4 kg at 10 years, (Lee, et al., 2001). The outcomes of these studies suggest that Japanese women have translated their body image into their weight status. After increasing their weight during pregnancy, many Japanese mothers then undertake activities to regain their pre-pregnancy body weight and shape just after birth, as they seek to achieve their ideal body image of being slim. Their opinions about their desired body image in the postpartum period are influenced by their exposure to media stereotypes (Slevec & Tiggemann, 2010; van den Berg et al., 2007).

The media, including newspapers, publicize in a sensational way how celebrity mothers change their body shape after birth, mostly emphasizing how quickly they regain their pre-pregnancy shape as they seek to become slim again (Roth, Homer, & Fenwick, 2011). The postpartum body shape of celebrity women, such as well-known actresses, is promoted in the media as the 'ideal' body shape of postpartum women. Many Japanese women are influenced by the media and seek to achieve the 'ideal' shape portrayed in the newspapers and magazines as their view of reality and give a priority to their weight and body shape. In addition, these media stereotype portrayals have influenced the opinions of males, peers, and family members about women's ideal body shape. A study by Swami et al. (2006) compared men's opinions about women's physical attractiveness between Britain and Japan, and found that Japanese men preferred a smaller BMI in women and considered BMI to be a more important factor in physical attractiveness for women than their British counterparts (Swami, et al., 2006). Japanese men were more likely to be swayed towards their opinions by the media and thus Japanese women, are very concerned about what other people, including Japanese men, think of them. There is also concern about the health consequences for infants of insufficient gestational weight gain in Japan, where weight gain is often limited to below 10 kg. (M. Inoue & Binns, 2012; H. Watanabe et al., 2010). Restricted gestational weight gain might be related to women's body image, but further studies are needed to clarify this association. However, a number of studies have found that Japanese women's body image has influenced their dieting behavior during pregnancy. A Japanese study of 248 pregnant women at an average of 28.6 gestational weeks (SD = 8.6) found that more than 35% were currently on a diet, including skipping meals more than three times a week although nearly 95% of participants in this study were in either the " underweight" or "normal" BMI categories (Takimoto, Mitsuishi, & Kato, 2011).

3. The Himeji-city Study of Postpartum Women's Body Image and Breastfeeding Outcomes

A study of the perceptions of postpartum Japanese women about their return to pre-pregnancy weight and their body image, particularly the level of concern about body appearance, was undertaken in Himeji City, Hyogo prefecture, which is located in central Japan, in 2007. This cross-sectional study used a structured and self-administered questionnaire that included the Attention to Body Shape scale (ABS) (Beebe, 1995). The study participants were all mothers aged between 16 and 45 years who were recruited at the health examinations offered to all infants and mothers at 18 months postpartum by the local government authorities in Japan. When the Himeji City Health Department sent an invitation letter for the 18 months health examination, the participants were asked to become involved in the study and to complete the questionnaire. Mothers, who were willing to participate in our study, brought the questionnaire with them when they brought their infants for their health examinations.. A total of 2,345 mothers were eligible to participate and 1,623 completed the questionnaire (response rate: 69.2%). For the final analysis, 1,612 questionnaires were used, due to missing data. Ethics approval for the study was obtained from the Human Research Ethics Committee of Curtin University and the Himeji City health authorities. The mean age of the mothers was 32.2 years (range from 18 to 44), and 56% of them were multiparous. Almost all were married (96.3%) and their husbands had regular jobs (99.9%). The majority of women were housewives (72.8%) and approximately 15% of them had delivered by Caesarean section. The LBW rate was 8.4% and 12% were regular smokers. In this study, the classification of BMI for adults, developed by the Japanese government in 2006, was used. Most women (75.4%) were in the 'normal' category of BMI (18.5-24.9), while 'underweight' (< 18.5) and 'obese' (25.0 ≤) were 19.6% and 5.0%, respectively. Mean pre-pregnancy BMI was 20.4 kg/m^2 (SD = 2.6). More than 42% of the mothers stated that they had not returned to their pre-pregnancy weight by 18 months postpartum. Approximately 18% were in the 'underweight (BMI < 18.5)' category. Nearly 60% of women had returned to their pre-pregnancy weight within six months after birth. The average weight that postpartum women retained at 18 months postpartum was 1.51 kg (SD = 0.42 for primipara (n = 652)) compared with their pre-pregnancy weight. In a multivariate analysis, maternal pre-pregnancy BMI was significantly associated with women's perceptions of their weight returning to the level before their first pregnancy (See Table 2). The results showed that even if their pre-pregnancy BMI was in the 'underweight' or 'normal', they tended not to perceive that their weight had returned to its pre-pregnancy level ($p < 0.01$). Regardless of their BMI levels, Japanese women were still concerned about their weight status after delivery. The respondents were asked about whether 'breastfeeding facilitated their efforts to regain their pre-pregnant body figure faster than infant formula' and more than 50% agreed with this statement. However, it is important to note that no significant association was found with the duration of 'any breastfeeding'. This result indicated that the Japanese women seem to have stronger expectations about the effects of breastfeeding on their efforts to return to pre-pregnancy weight.

In this study, postpartum women's body image was assessed using the Attention to the Body Shape scale (ABS) (Beebe, 1995). The ABS is a seven-item assessment tool containing statements about the individual's perceptions of body shape and appearance. Each item was rated on a five-point Likert scale ranging from 1 = definitely disagree to 5 = definitely agree. The total scores ranged from 7 to 35 and the higher the score, the higher the level of consciousness about the individual's body shape. In a recent study, a Japanese version of the ABS was verified for internal consistency (α = 0.70-0.80) (Kagawa, 2004). A value of Cronbach's alpha level of internal consistency above 0.7 indicates a high reliability, between 0.5 and 0.7 shows moderate, 0.2 to 0.4 is fair, and below 0.2 means a low reliability (Nunnally & Bernstein, 1994). The results of the ABS in the Himeji study are shown in Table 4. The average score of the ABS was 24.2 (SD = 4.2). Women in the Himeji study were conscious about their body shape at a level higher than Beebe's study,(in the USA) ranging from 23.9 (SD = 4.4) to 24.1 (SD = 4.1), (Beebe, 1995) but slightly lower than the Kagawa's study by 24.9 (SD = 3.5) (Kagawa, Uchida, Uenishi, Binns, & Hills, 2007). While the sample size and characteristics of Kagawa's study was different from the Himeji study, there is an indication that the Japanese women's body image, particularly consciousness about body shape has been retained from pre-pregnancy to postpartum periods. More than two thirds (65.9%) in this study disagreed with the statement that they were 'not self-consciousness about their body shape' and more than half (55.4%) agreed that they were 'attentive to their body shape'. (Note the wording of item 3 in the ABS is a as a double-negative and therefore most of the Japanese respondents were self-conscious about their body shape). The same percentage of the respondents (54.1%) also stated that they considered buying particular clothes in order to cover weaker points of their body shape. The majority answered most items with either 'strongly agree'/'agree' or 'neutral'. The Cronbach alpha level for the ABS was 0.80, which shows a high level of internal consistency and was higher than the original study of 49 US women reported by Beebe (1995) ranging from 0.70 to 0.78 and a study by Kagawa et al. (2007) using 139 single, non-lactating Japanese women at 0.70.

However, the ABS score was not directly associated with 'breastfeeding' to six months in the binary logistic regression model (adjusted OR = 0.95, 95% CI = 0.90-1.01). While the total ABS score was not associated with breastfeeding, an additional question on "perceptions of breast shape changes due to lactation" in the Himeji study was significantly associated with the duration of any breastfeeding to six months (adjusted OR = 0.60, 95% CI = 0.40-0.91) (Madoka. Inoue, 2012).

Table 2. Factors associating with the postpartum women's perceptions of weight return to pregnancy level (backwards stepwise regression n = 1,612)

Factors	Adjusted OR	95% CI
Respondents' BMI before the first pregnancy		
< 18.5	**0.14**	**0.04-0.42**
18.5-24.9	**0.37**	**0.12-0.99**
≥ 25	1.00	Reference

-2 Log likelihood = 976.287.

Non-significant factors (potential confounders) included in the full model were mothers' age, ABS score, any breastfeeding duration.

Table 3. The Attention to Body Shape Scale (ABS) among participants in the Himeji study (n = 1,612)

Item	Strong Agree (%)	Agree (%)	Neutral (%)	Disagree (%)	Strong Disagree (%)
I place great importance of deal with body shape	4.3	36.6	36.1	15.0	8.0
I buy a product that promise to give me a better body	4.7	40.7	38.7	11.0	4.9
I am not self-conscious about my body shape	1.6	7.4	25.1	42.6	23.3
I am always trying to improve my body shape	9.8	44.3	36.2	7.4	2.3
I wear clothes that highlight best aspect of my body and hide the worst aspect of my body	8.7	48.5	34.8	6.5	1.6
It really bothers me when I cannot keep my body in shape	8.1	42.1	34.0	12.9	2.8
I am very attentive to my body shape	6.1	49.6	34.7	8.1	1.5

As these measures are based on self-reports, over or under estimation of body weight may have occurred and body image is always subjective. Several studies have found that Japanese women often over estimate their weight (Ayumi. Sugawara et al., 2010). The likelihood is that this data may therefore over estimate actual weights. In the Himeji study 233 participants (14.5%) engaged in activities to regain their body shape. The most common activity was to wear a special bra or underwear, which was usually started within one to two months postpartum. They also undertook other activities including having a low calorie and low fat diet and increased exercise time designed to regain their body shape. Overall, Japanese postpartum women were very focused on their body shape and weight status.

4. Discussion

In Japan, a combination of 'women's desire to be slim', media stereotypes of the 'ideal' women's shape, and inappropriate weight gain during pregnancy has encouraged mothers to mainly focus on their postpartum body shape and weight status with little attention to breastfeeding benefits. The results of the Himeji-city study suggested a strong consciousness of body shape and weight status among Japanese postpartum women. The total ABS score and women's perceptions of weight return to their pre-pregnancy levels were not significantly related to the duration of 'any breastfeeding' at six months post-partum. However women's perceptions of breast shape changes were significantly associated with 'any breastfeeding' at six months postpartum in the Himeji-city study. This suggests that further studies are needed to improve the ABS for use in the Japanese culture.

The average weight retention after pregnancy of Japanese women is smaller than in other Asian counties. In a cross-sectional study of 97 postpartum women in Korea, Kwon et al (2004) found that they retained on average 1.87 kg (SD = 3.83) additional weight at one year postpartum. This study found that a higher pre-pregnancy BMI ($\geq$ 23 kg/m^2), greater weight gain during pregnancy, and family monthly income are factors that significantly influence weight retention in postpartum women. As Japanese women are relatively smaller pre-pregnancy with a lower BMI and have less weight gain during pregnancy than other Asian countries, their postpartum weight retention would be lower (M. Inoue & Binns, 2013). However, Japanese women have a strong desire to be slim and this is at the same level pre- and post- pregnancy and therefore makes efforts to regain their body shape and pre-pregnancy weight status regardless of the length of breastfeeding. The long-term desire of Japanese women to be slim influences the rate of weight retention. A prospective cohort study by Lyu et al (2009) showed that the average weight retention in Taiwanese women (n = 122) was 1.32 kg (SD = 3.99) at one year postpartum. Although breastfeeding duration was not associated with 1-year postpartum weight retention in this study, increased energy intake, energy consumption per kg and decreased physical activities were more likely to influence weight changes at 1 year postpartum at 50-60% (Lyu, et al., 2009). Moreover, Japanese women have been conditioned to have an ideal body image of being slim since they are young. A study of 18,512 university students from 22 countries, examined attitudes to weight status in five regions, Asia Pacific, Central and Eastern Europe, the Mediterranean, South America, and North-Western Europe and United State (US). This study showed that Japanese women had the highest prevalence of perceived overweight (63%, 95% CI = 57-68) among all 22 countries surveyed (Wardle, Haase, & Steptoe, 2006). Since Japanese women have established a strong body image of 'being slim' as their ideal, education for infant feeding must be related to an understanding of women's body image, especially for programs directed towards the younger generations. For the majority of women, their body image perceptions during pregnancy and in the postpartum period are based on the attitudes which are formed pre-pregnancy (Chang, Chao, & Kenney, 2006). Breastfeeding education directed towards young and pregnant women is essential to enable them to understand the importance of establishing appropriate body image, knowledge, and attitudes towards infant feeding practices.

Similarly the body image of women in the postpartum period is strongly related to body image during their pregnancy or before their pregnancy. Women's body image during pregnancy is also known to affect decisions on infant feeding methods. In Taiwan, a study of 195 women at 28 weeks gestation explored relationships between body image, maternal-infant attachment, and infant feeding methods (Huang, Wang, & Chen, 2004). The results of this study showed that women with a poor self-image of their body found it difficult to relate to their fetus, after they became pregnant. Consequently, women who had a negative body image during pregnancy tended to choose bottle feeding as it was harder for them to establish maternal-infant attachment (Huang, et al., 2004). An English study of how women's concerns about their body shape and weight changes contributed to the intention of breastfeeding (n = 12,000) found that the women who were preoccupied with their body shape were less likely to intend breastfeeding their infant (Barnes, Stein, Smith, & Pollock, 1997).

The issue of body image in postpartum women deserves more attention from health professionals and authorities. While several studies have reported that Asian women are more sensitive about their weight status and body shape, there are a few studies that included psychological/cultural factors including women's body image (Cheng, et al., 2011; Fukuoka, Ueoka, Koya, & Ishii, 2012). Body image is important and also impacts on issues such as depression. An Australian cohort study of 116 pregnant women investigated their body dissatisfaction and depression levels throughout pregnancy to 12 month postpartum and found that they were most likely to have negative feelings about body weight and shape at six months postpartum (Clark, Skouteris, Wertheim, Paxton, & Milgrom, 2009). In this study body image, including feelings of 'being fatter' and perceptions of changes in weight and body shape were worse in all postpartum periods (six weeks, six months, and 12 months postpartum), than throughout their pregnancy (17-21 weeks gestation and 32-35 weeks gestation) (Clark, et al., 2009). Likewise, the level of body dissatisfaction was significantly related to greater weight and worse mental health status at nine months postpartum in a prospective cohort study of 506 postpartum women in the Unites States (Gjerdingen et al., 2009). In this study, women retained their weight at 9 months postpartum with 2.5 kg (SD = 7.1) in average (Gjerdingen, et al., 2009). However, postpartum women still need to be encouraged and educated to continue breastfeeding in order to gain maximum benefit from breastfeeding. Cultural/psychological factors including women's body image are important when considering breastfeeding outcomes in Japan.

CONCLUSION

This chapter has discussed postpartum weight retention and women's body image and their association with breastfeeding outcomes in Japan. Japanese postpartum women are very conscious about their body shape and weight status, and this consciousness about their beauty originates pre-pregnancy or even earlier. Body image was assessed using the Attention to the Body Shape Scale (ABS) and showed that Japanese women are very conscious of their body shape at 18 months postpartum.

Postpartum weight retention is less in Japanese women than in other Asian and Western countries. While there are many studies that have examined breastfeeding outcomes, there have been few studies that have included psychological and cultural factors, including women's body image. There is an association between concern over breast shape and the duration of breastfeeding, with mothers who express this concern having a shorter duration of breastfeeding. There is a tension between this belief and the understanding of many Japanese mothers that breastfeeding will promote postpartum weight loss. Asian women, particularly Japanese, are more focused on their body shape and weight status, and these factors deserve more attention in studies of factors associated with breastfeeding outcomes, other infant feeding practices and postpartum weight loss. This information would be useful in developing breastfeeding promotion programs.

The average postpartum weight retention of Japanese women after pregnancy was lower than for other Asian countries and this may be related to their perceptions of body image and their desire to return to their pre-pregnancy weight.

References

Baker, J. L., Gamborg, M., Heitmann, B. L., Lissner, L., Sorensen, T. I., & Rasmussen, K. M. (2008). Breastfeeding reduces postpartum weight retention. *Am J Clin Nutr, 88*(6), 1543-1551. doi:10.3945/ajcn.2008. 263 79.

Barnes, J., Stein, A., Smith, T., & Pollock, J. I. (1997). Extreme attitudes to body shape, social and psychological factors and a reluctance to breast feed. ALSPAC Study Team. Avon Longitudinal Study of Pregnancy and Childhood. *Journal of the Royal Society of Medicine 90*(10), 551-559.

Beebe, D. W. (1995). The attention to body shape scale: A new measure of body focus. *Journal of Personality Assessment, 65*(3), 486-501.

Chang, S. R., Chao, Y. M., & Kenney, N. J. (2006). I am a woman and i'm pregnant: Body image of women in Taiwan during the third trimester of pregnancy. *Birth, 33*(2), 147-153. doi: BIR087 [pii]10.1111/j.0730-7659. 2006.00087.x.

Cheng, H. R., Walker, L. O., Tseng, Y. F., & Lin, P. C. (2011). Post-partum weight retention in women in Asia: a systematic review. [Review]. *Obes Rev, 12*(10), 770-780. doi: 10.1111/j.1467-789X.2011.00886.x.

Clark, A., Skouteris, H., Wertheim, E. H., Paxton, S. J., & Milgrom, J. (2009). The relationship between depression and body dissatisfaction across pregnancy and the postpartum: a prospective study. *J Health Psychol, 14*(1), 27-35. doi: 14/1/27 [pii]10.1177/1359105308097940.

Drewnowski, A. (2000). Nutrition transition and global dietary trends. [Review]. *Nutrition, 16*(7-8), 486-487.

Fukuoka, Y., Ueoka, H., Koya, N. F., Y., & Ishii, M. (2012). Anthropometric Method for Determining Masked Obesity in the Young Japanese Female Population. *Journal of Anthropology, 2012*, 5. doi:10.1155/ 2012/ 595614.

Gjerdingen, D., Fontaine, P., Crow, S., McGovern, P., Center, B., & Miner, M. (2009). Predictors of mothers' postpartum body dissatisfaction. *Women & Health, 49*(6), 491-504. doi: 917670608 [pii]10.1080/036302409034239 98.

Hayashi, F., Takimoto, H., Yoshita, K., & Yoshiike, N. (2006). Perceived body size and desire for thinness of young Japanese women: a population-based survey. *Br J Nutr, 96*(6), 1154-1162. doi: S0007114507207603 [pii].

Herring, S. J., Rich-Edwards, J. W., Oken, E., Rifas-Shiman, S. L., Kleinman, K. P., & Gillman, M. W. (2008). Association of postpartum depression with weight retention 1 year after childbirth. [Research Support, N. I. H., Extramural Research Support, Non-U.S. Gov't]. *Obesity, 16*(6), 1296-1301. doi: 10. 1038/oby.2008.71.

Huang, H. C., Wang, S. Y., & Chen, C. H. (2004). Body image, maternal-fetal attachment, and choice of infant feeding method: A study in Taiwan. *Birth, 31*(3), 183-188.

Inoue, M. (2012). *Breastfeeding and perceptions of breast shape changes in Australian and Japanese women.* PhD PhD dissatation, Curtin University, Perth.

Inoue, M., & Binns, C. (2012). *Breastfeeding and perceptions of breast shape changes in Australian and Japanese women (in press).* Saarbrücken, Germany: LAP_LAMBERT.

Inoue, M., & Binns, C. (2013). Maternal Body Mass Index and weight gain during pregnancy in Asia *Maternity: Perspectives, Challenges and Social Implication.* Hauppauge, NY: Nova Science Publishers Inc.

Kac, G., Benicio, M. H., Velasquez-Melendez, G., Valente, J. G., & Struchiner, C. J. (2004). Breastfeeding and postpartum weight retention in a cohort of Brazilian women. [Research Support, Non-U. S. Gov't]. *Am J Clin Nutr, 79*(3), 487-493.

Kagawa, M. (2004). *Ethnic and cultural influences on body composition, lifestyle and body image among males.* PhD PhD dissatation, Curtin University of Technology, Perth.

Kagawa, M., Uchida, H., Uenishi, K., Binns, C., & Hills, A. P. (2007). Applicability of the Ben-Tovim Walker Body Attitudes Questionnaire (BAQ) and the Attention to Body Shape Scale (ABS) in Japanese Males and Females. *Eating behaviors,* 8(3), 277-284.

Kwon, J. H., Lee, S. H., Lee, P. R., & Park, H. S. (2004). Factors Associated with Weight Gain at 1 Year Postpartum. *J Korean Acad Fam Med,* 25(9), 661-668.

Lee, J. S., Kawakubo, K., Kobayashi, Y., Mori, K., Kasihara, H., & Tamura, M. (2001). Effects of ten year body weight variability on cardiovascular risk factors in Japanese middle-aged men and women. *Int J Obes Relat Metab Disord,* 25(7), 1063-1067. doi: 10.1038/sj.ijo.0801633.

Lyu, L. C., Lo, C. C., Chen, H. F., Wang, C. Y., & Liu, D. M. (2009). A prospective study of dietary intakes and influential factors from pregnancy to postpartum on maternal weight retention in Taipei, Taiwan. *British journal of nutrition,* 102(12), 1828.

Minister of Health Labour and Walfare. (2011). *The 2010 National Survey of Child Growth* (Article in Japanese). Tokyo: Minister of Health Labour and Walfare Retrieved from http://www.mhlw.go.jp/stf/houdou/2r985200 0001t3so.html.

Ministry of Health Labour and Walfare. (2002). *The 2000 National Nutritional Survey* (in Japanese). Tokyo: Ministry of Health Labour and Walfare.

Ministry of Health Labour and Welfare. (2009). *The 2008 Natioal Nutritional Survey* (in Japanese). Tokyo: Ministry of Health Labour and Welfare, Retrieved from http://www.mhlw.go.jp/houdou/2009/11/h1109-1.html.

Ministry of Health Labour and Welfare. (2010). *The 2009 National Health and Nutritional Survey* (in Japanese). Tokyo: Ministry of Health Labour and Walfare, Retrieved from http:// www.mhlw.go.jp/bunya/kenkou/kenkou_ eiyou_chousa.html.

Montgomery, K. S., Bushee, T. D., Phillips, J. D., Kirkpatrick, T., Catledge, C., Braveboy, K., Douglas, G. M. (2011). Women's challenges with postpartum weight loss. *Matern Child Health J* 15(8), 1176-1184. doi: 10.1007/s10995-010-0681-9.

Nunnally, J. C., & Bernstein, I. H. (1994). *Psychometric theory* (3rd edition ed.). New York New York : McGraw-Hill.

Popkin, B. M. (2004). The nutrition transition: an overview of world patterns of change. [Research Support, U. S. Gov't, P. H. S.Review]. *Nutr Rev, 62* (7 Pt 2), S140-143.

Roth, H., Homer, C., & Fenwick, J. (2011). 'Bouncing back': How Australia's leading women's magazines portray the postpartum 'body'. *Women Birth*. doi: S1871-5192(11)00207-1 [pii]10.1016/j.wombi.2011.08.004.

Slevec, J., & Tiggemann, M. (2010). Attitudes towards cosmetic surgery in middle-aged women: Body image, aging anxiety and the media. *Psychology of women quarterly, 34*(1), 65-74. doi: 10.1111/j.1471-6402. 2009. 01542.x.

Sugawara, A., Saito, K., Sato, M., Kodama, S., & Sone, H. (2009). Thinness in Japanese young women. *Epidemiology, 20*(3), 464-465. doi: 10.1097/ EDE.0b013e31819ed4ed00001648-200905000-00028 [pii].

Sugawara, A., Yanagishita, J., Sano, A., Wong, Y., NT Le, D. S., Martin, J., Sone, H. (2010). Body Image: International Comparisons: From the Symposium Held at the 15th International Congress of Dietetics. *Nutrition Today, 45*(3), 113-117. doi: 10.1097/NT.0b013e3181dec6bb.

Swami, V., Caprario, C., Tovée, M. J., & Furnham, A. (2006). Female physical attractiveness in Britain and Japan: a cross-cultural study. *European Journal of Personality, 20*(1), 69-81. doi: 10.1002/per.568.

Takimoto, H., Mitsuishi, C., & Kato, N. (2011). Attitudes toward pregnancy related changes and self-judged dieting behavior. *Asia Pac J Clin Nutr, 20*(2), 212-219.

van den Berg, P., Paxton, S. J., Keery, H., Wall, M., Guo, J., & Neumark-Sztainer, D. (2007). Body dissatisfaction and body comparison with media images in males and females. *Body Image, 4*(3), 257-268. doi: S1740-1445(07)00043-5 [pii]10.1016/j.bodyim.2007.04.003.

Wardle, J., Haase, A. M., & Steptoe, A. (2006). Body image and weight control in young adults: international comparisons in university students from 22 countries. *Int J Obes (Lond), 30*(4), 644-651. doi: 0803050 [pii] 10.1038/sj.ijo.0803050.

Watanabe, E., Lee, J. s., Kawakubo, K., & Marui, E. (2008). Correlation between change in body weight and lifestyle behaviour before and after childbirth (in Japanese). *Minzoku Eisei, 74*(1), 3-12.

Watanabe, H., Inoue, K., Doi, M., Matsumoto, M., Ogasawara, K., Fukuoka, H., & Nagai, Y. (2010). Risk factors for term small for gestational age infants in women with low pre-pregnancy body mass index. *J Obstet Gynaecol Res, 36*(3), 506-512. doi: JOG1170 [pii]10.1111/j.1447-0756. 2010.01170.x.

Word Health Organization. (2011). *WHO Global InfoBase: International Comparisons* Retrieved 28. January, 2013, from https://apps.who.int/infobase/Comparisons.aspx.

Yoshiike, N., Kaneda, F., & Takimoto, H. (2002). Epidemiology of obesity and public health strategies for its control in Japan. *Asia Pac J Clin Nutr, 11 Suppl 8*, S727-731.

In: Weight Gain
Editors: A. Pirotte and T. Libert ISBN: 978-1-62618-800-6

Chapter 4

CAN EXERCISE TRAINING REDUCE THE PREVALENCE OF OBESITY WITH FAT DIET?

Naziha El Elj[1]*, Gérard Lac[2], Monia Zaouali[3], Zouhair Tabka[3], Abdelaziz Kammoun[1], Najoua Gharbi[1] and Saloua El Fezaa[1]

[1]Laboratory of Animal Physiology, Department of Biology, Faculty of Sciences of Tunis, Campus Universitaire, Tunis, Tunisia
[2]Laboratory of Physiology, Motor Performance, University B. Pascal, Bat Biology B, The Cézeaux, Aubière, France
[3]Physiology Laboratory and Function Tests, Faculty of Medicine Ibn El Jazzar, Sousse, Tunisia

ABSTRACT

High-fat diet induces obesity. It is considered as the second most lethal habit after smoking. The purpose of this study was to examine the effect of exercise training on the control of weight gain in rats receiving fat diet.

* Corresponding author: Dr Naziha El Elj. Address : Laboratoire de Physiologie Animale, Département de Biologie, Faculté des Sciences de Tunis, Campus Universitaire, 1060 Tunis, Tunisie. Tel: 00216 71 87 26 00 - 00216 97 38 98 13; Fax: 00216 71 88 54 80; E-mail: naziha_elj@yahoo.fr.

The study was carried out with three groups of rats (n=12); the standard diet sedentary group (SS) (control group), standard diet with exercise (SE) and high fat diet with exercise (FE). Animals in high fat diet group were fed a diet containing 10% olive oil (weight/weight). Trained rats swam 1 hour/day 5 times weekly for 4 weeks.

Significant reductions in weight gain and in food intake were observed with training ($p<0.001$). Body weight was maintained in trained rats receiving fat diet. Fat diet significantly increased both insulin concentrations ($p<0.05$), glycaemia ($p<0.001$) and muscle glycogen ($p<0.001$).

This research demonstrated the efficient effect of exercise training on preventing overweight in rats fed fat diet. Our results showed, as well, the positive effect of physical exercise on reducing both food intake and weight gain.

Keywords: Fat diet, Body weight, Exercise training, rats

INTRODUCTION

Obesity and overweight have in the last decade become a global problem. According to the World Health Organization (WHO) back in 2005 approximately 1.6 billion adults over the age of 15 years were overweight, at least 400 million adults were obese and at least 20 million children under the age of 5 years were overweight.

The scale of the obesity problem has a number of serious consequences for individuals and government health systems. In fact, obesity is a risk factor for heart disease, several cancers, hypertension, diabetes, arthritis, and multiple sclerosis (Birse et al. 2010; Astrup et al., 2005). In addition to being hazardous to health, obesity is also an economic handicap.

It is obvious now that high fat diet causes obesity (Shai et al. 2008, hanricsson et al. 1995). Therefore, it is a problem mainly in countries with high fat diets. The increased consumption of energy-dense foods such as those high in fat and the lack of physical activity are the two main ways leading to obesity.

Actually, strategies recommended for weight control have generally included healthy diets and physical exercise (Shai et al. 2008, hanricsson et al. 1995).

Physical exercise can prevent weight gain mainly because it lowers the energetic balance by increasing energy expenditure as it was reported in studies on wheel running rats (Levin et al., 2004; Bi et al., 2005). In addition, physical activity also improves blood lipidic constants, especially HDL cholesterol (Ben Ounis et al., 2008), as lipid oxidation is the major form of energy generation during moderate and prolonged exercises (Gomes et al., 2004).

Besides, it seems to be easier, for most people, to maintain regular physical activity than to deprive them of their favorite foods, if it is only to prevent overweight. Therefore, the aim of the present study was to examine the effect of exercise training on the control of weight gain in rats receiving high fat diet.

Methods and Materials

Animals and Treatments

Male albino Wistar rats weighing 130-150g obtained from SIPHAT (Tunis, Tunisia) were used in this study. Before any experiment, all animals were kept for 1 week in the same laboratory conditions of temperature (22±2°C), relative humidity (70±4%), and a 12h light/dark cycle. They received a nutritionally standard diet (SICO, Sfax, Tunisia) and tap water. All experiments were carried out with the approval of the local animal use committee.

Animals were randomly divided into three groups of 12 rats: the standard diet sedentary group (SS) (control group), standard diet with exercise (SE) (62% carbohydrate, 17% protein, 4% fat; 352 Kcal) and high-fat diet with exercise (FE) (56% carbohydrate, 15% protein, 14% fat; 407 Kcal).

Experimental Protocol

Food intake and animals weight were measured every day. Animals in the trained groups were subjected to swimming exercise in groups of 6 rats in a swimming tank of 100×50 cm with a depth of 50 cm, filled with tap water. The water temperature was kept at 32±2°C. The trained groups swam 1 h/day 5 times weekly for 4 wks. During 5 days before the experiment, the animals were acclimated to the water and exercise with a gradual increase in swimming period. All animals were sacrificed by decapitation 24 h after the last bout of exercise.

Blood was collected into dry tubes and centrifuged at 3000g for 15 min at 25°C to separate serum. After blood collection, the entire muscle of both paws were dissected out and immediately immersed in 0.9 % NaCl solution. Glucose concentration was immediately measured. All samples were stored frozen at -30°C until the time for analysis.

Determination of Hormonal and Biochemical Parameters

Corticosterone and Insulin concentrations were determined using specific radioimmunoassay kits for the determination on the hormones in rat serum (DSL-Texas-USA). Plasma glucose and triglyceride were measured by colorimetric methods using commercial kits obtained from BIOMAGHREB (Tunis, Tunisia).

Muscle glycogen was determined immediately after the sacrifice using the method of Good et al. (1933).

Statistical Analysis

Results are expressed as mean ±SE. A two-way ANOVA was performed for effects of diet and physical activity on each variable. Statistical comparisons between groups were done by Student t test. Significance was accepted at the level of $p<0.05$.

Results

At the end of the study, exercised animals with and without fat diet had a lower weight gain than did sedentary group ($P < 0.001$, Table 1). Weight gain was higher in trained rats receiving fat diet in comparison with standard diet (FE vs. SE; $P < 0.001$, Table 1). Food intake was lower in trained rats with different diets ($P < 0.001$, Table 1). Corticosterone levels increased significantly with training (SE vs. SS; $P < 0.05$, Figure 1). Rats fed high-fat diet have higher insulin ($P < 0.05$, Figure 2), glycaemia ($P < 0.001$, Table 1), and muscle glycogen levels ($P < 0.01$, Table 1). Plasma triglycerides were decreased in trained groups ($P < 0.05$, Table 1).

Table 1. Values Means ±SE of food intake, weight gain, glycaemia, muscle glycogen and triglyceridemia in different groups of rats

	SS	SE	FE
Food intake (g /day)	15.86±0.2	13.86±0.2[a]	14.6±0.1[a]
Food intake (kcal/day)	55,67±1.05	48,47±0.05[a]	56,93±0.75[b]
Weight gain/30d (g)	89.96±3.3	67.86±3.4[a]	77.56±2.3[a b]
Glycaemia (g/l)	1.16±0.03	1.16±0.04	1.66±0.05[a b]
Muscle glycogen (g/100g)	3.6±0.5	2.46±0.2	4.16±0.2[a b]
Plasma triglycerides (mmol/l)	1.76±0.2	1.08±0.17[a]	1.16±0.16[a]

[a] Significantly different from group SS; [b] significantly different from group SE.

Discussion

The objective of this study was to investigate the effects of endurance exercise training on beating overweight induced with fat diet.

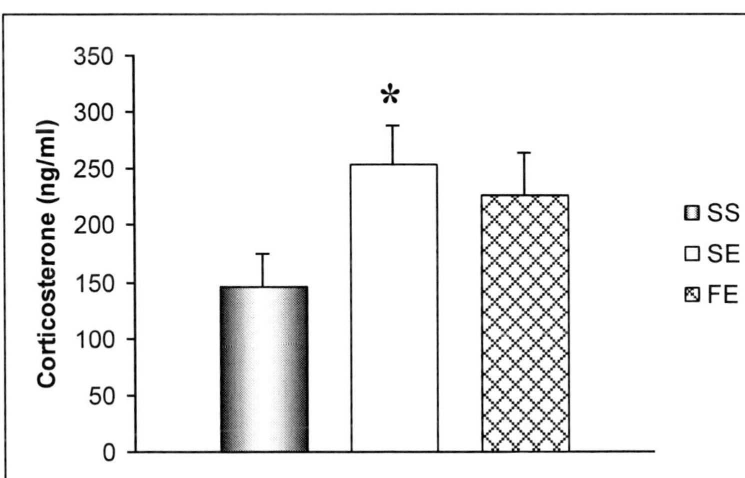

Figure 1. Effect of physical training and fat dietary on corticosterone concentrations. Values are mean±SE. * $p<0.05$ (SE vs. SS).

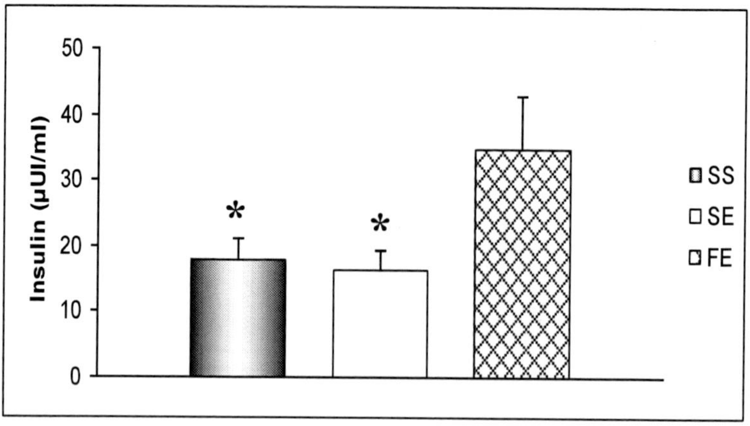

Figure 2. Effect of physical training and fat dietary on insulin concentrations. Values are mean±SE. * $p<0.05$ (SS and SE vs. FE).

As a main result of this research, we showed that 30 days of endurance training induced significant lower weight gain and food intake even with fat diet. Similarly, Mathey et al. (2000) and Ebal et al. (2007) revealed decreased weight gain and food intake during 5 weeks of moderate strength exercise. The decreased body weight in trained rats may be explained by the reduced fat mass as result of exercise training (Ebal et al., 2007; Mathey et al. 2000). Moreover, it may result, also, from the negative energy balance linked with increased energy expenditure during the exercise (Bi et al., 2005) and decreased food intake. Physical training, generally, results in less weight gain independently of the diet used; the negative energy balance alone is responsible for weight reduction (Levin et al., 2004; Bi et al., 2005).

In addition, high-fat diet results showed that body weight was lower in trained rat receiving fat diet in comparison with control (sedentary group with standard diet) and higher in comparison with trained group with standard diet. This demonstrated the important role of exercise training in the attenuation of increased body weight following a high-fat diet. Actually, it was demonstrated that high-fat low-carbohydrate diets were used to enhance weight loss (Ebal et al., 2007; Sacks et al., 2009).

Besides, it has been demonstrated that high-fat diet leads to hypophagia, probably due to an adaptation faculty developed by animals with regard to energy value of the diet and not according to the quantity ingested in mass. This can explain the decreased food intake observed in fat-diet rats (Ebal et al., 2007).

In our study, corticosterone levels increased in response to exercise training. In fact, it was reported that periods of substantially increased volume or intensity training increase cortisol secretion in humans (Izquierdo et al., 2006), thereby indicating this hormone to be useful marker of chronic strength training stress (Kraemer et al., 2005). The increased levels of corticosterone observed in this study is consistent with the study of Izquierdo et al. (2006) and Ebal et al. (2007), who showed, similarly, increased levels of corticosterone in rats following training. Actually, this hormone can interfere with food intake regulation (Gotoh et al., 2005) because corticoids were shown to inhibit ghrelin production, which is known to stimulate food intake (Proulx et al., 2005). Therefore, we may propose that the training regime applied to the rats reduced food intake through a feedback loop between corticosterone and ghrelin level. Such an activation of the hypothalamo-hypophyso-adrenal axis (HHAA) with an anorexigen effect has been reported in the wheel-running model rat (Burden et al., 1993; De Rijke et al., 2005), in particular an elevation of the CRF expression and/or the decrease of NPY expression (Bi S. et al., 2005).

We haven't recorded any significant alteration in carbohydrate metabolism parameters in response to exercise training, neither in insulin, nor in glycaemia, nor in muscle glycogen. This can be explained by the endurance type of training. In fact, it was demonstrated that regular endurance training leads to a multitude of metabolic adaptations in skeletal muscle that result in a decreased use of carbohydrates and a concomitant increase in fat oxidation and lipid use as energetic substrate during exercise (Melanson et al., 2009), which reduces changes in carbohydrate metabolism.

However, fat diet significantly increased glycaemia, insulinemia and muscle glycogen which disrupt overall metabolism. It has been reported that adaptation to high-fat diet change substrate utilization toward high fat oxidation during exercise (Jahreis et al., 1991). Several mechanisms have been demonstrated that could account for this change, specially decreased muscle glycogen utilization during exercise (Lapachet et al., 1996) leads to glycogen accumulation in muscle. Indeed, it had been demonstrated that a high-fat diet attenuates the decrease in liver glycogen storage and totally abolishes the decrease in muscle glycogen storage and possibly utilization during exercise (Helge et al., 1998). Moreover, we noted that plasma levels of glucose and insulin were significantly increased by fat-diet in spite of training. This was consistent with other studies. For example, it has been demonstrated in humans that endurance training did not significantly affect glucose production (Coggan et al., 1995), and treadmill training in rats has been reported to have no effect in resting glucose levels (Donova et al., 1990). Thus, unchanged levels of glucose would not produce any alteration in insulin concentrations in this state. Nevertheless, our results showed that glucose and insulin concentrations were significantly increased by the high-fat diet. It has been demonstrated that fat-rich diet affect the substrate recruitment, and most likely oxidation with a preferential mobilization and oxidation of fatty acids (FA) rather than carbohydrate oxidation (Helge et al., 1996). In addition, it has been shown that high-fat diet increased glucose production by reducing insulin suppression of glucose appearance and by increasing the gluconeogenesis (Gobzalez-Manchon et al., 1989). Accordingly, plasma levels of glucose increased without being altered by oxidation. This might increase insulin production in order to regulate the glucose concentration in blood. Indeed, it has been demonstrated that chronic high-fat diet induces widespread insulin resistance (Liu et al., 1996). Thus, a diet high in fat is associated with decreased glucose tolerance and decreased insulin sensitivity in the whole body. Insulin resistance is a metabolic state when normal or high concentrations of insulin produce a less than normal bio-logical response (Liu et al., 1996). This insulin resistance induced by the high-fat diet was not corrected by physical exercise (Liu et al., 1996). This can explain the higher levels of glucose and insulin obtained with the fat diet.

We can conclude that endurance training protects against overweight induced by fat diets; first, by decreasing food intake, and second, by increasing energy expenditure. It seems to be effective in the fight against obesity.

REFERENCES

Astrup, A. (2005). The role of dietary fat in obesity. *Semin Vasc Med.* 5 (1), 40-47.

Ben Ounis, O., Elloumi, M., Ben Chiekh, I., Zbidi, A., Amri, M., Lac, G., & Tabka, Z. (2008). Effects of two-month physical-endurance and diet-restriction programmes on lipid profiles and insulin resistance in obese adolescent boys. *Diabetes & Metabolism*, 34, 595-600.

Bi, S., Scott, K. A., Hyun, J., Ladenheim, E. E., & Moran, T. H. (2005). Running wheel activity prevents hyperphagia and obesity in Otsuka long-evans Tokushima Fatty rats: Role of hypothalamic signalling. *Endocrinology*, *146*, 1676-1685.

Birse, R. T., Choi, J., Reardon, K., Rodriguez, J., Graham, S., Diop, S., Ocorr, K., Bodmer, R., Oldham, S. (2010). High-fat-diet-induced obesity and heart dysfunction are regulated by the TOR pathway in Drosophila. *Cell Metab,*12 (5), 533-544.

Bruden, V. R., White, B. D., Dean, R. G., & Martin, R. J. (1993). Activity of the hypothalamic-pituitary-adrenal axis is elevated in rats with activity-based anorexia. *Journal of Nutrition*, *123*, 1217- 1225.

Coggan, A. R., Swanson, S. C., Mendenhall, L. A., Habash, D. L. (1995). Effect of endurance training on hepatic glycogenolysis and gluconeogenesis during prolonged exercise in men. *Am J Physiol,* 31, 375-383.

De Rijke, C. E., Hillebrand, J. J., Verhagen, L. A., Roeling, T. A., & Adan, R. A. (2005). Hypothalamic neuropeptide expression following chronic food restriction in sedentary and wheel-running rats. *Journal of Molecular Endocrinology*, *35*, 381-390.

Donova, C. M., Sumida, K. D. (1990). Training improves glucose homeostasis in rats during exercise via glucose production. *Am J Physio,* 27, 770-776.

Ebal, E., Cavalie, H., Michaux, O., & Lac, G. (2007). Effect of a moderate exercise on the regulatory hormones of food intake in rats. *Appetite*, *49*, 521-524.

Ebal, E., Cavalié, H., Michaux, O., & Lac, G. (2007). Effect of a lipid-enriched diet on body composition and some regulatory hormones of food intake in growing rats. *Annales d'Endocrinologie*, *68*, 366-371.

Gobzalez-Manchon, C., Ayuso, M., Parrilla, R. (1989). Control of hepatic gluconeogenesis: role of fatty acid oxidation. *Arch Biochem Biophys*, 271, 1-9.

Gomes, M. R., Pires, I. S. O., De Castro, I. A., Tirapegui, J. (2004). Effect of moderate physical exercise on plasma and tissue levels of insulin-like growth factor-1 in adult rats. *Nutrition Research*, *24*, 555-564.

Good, C. A., Krames, H., & Somogyi, M. (1933). Chemical Procedures for analysis of poly saccharides. *Method in enzymalogy*, *VIII*, p.34.

Gotoh, K., Fukagawa, T., Fukagawa, T., Noguchi, H., Kakuma, T., Sakata, T., & Yochimatsu, H. (2005). Glucagon-like peptide 1, corticotrophin-releasing hormone, and hypothalamic neuronal histamine interact in the leptin-signaling pathway to regulate feeding behaviour. *The Federation of American Societies for Experimental Biology Journal*, *19*, 1131-1133.

Helge, J. W., Ayre, K., Chaunchaiyakul, S., Hulbert, A. J., Kiens, B. (1998). Interaction of training and diet on metabolism and endurance during exercise in man. *Journal of Applied Physiology*, 85, 1342-1348.

Helge, J. W., Richter, E. A. and Kiens, B. (1996). Interaction of training and diet on metabolism and endurance during exercise in man. *Journal of Applied Physiology*, 292, 293-306.

Henriksson, J. (1995). Influence of exercise on insulin sensitivity. *J Cardiovasc Risk*, *2*, 303-309.

Izquierdo, M., Ibanez, J., Gonzalez- Badillo, J. J., Hakkinen, K., Ratamess, N. A., Kraemer, W. J., French, D. N., Eslava, J., Altadill, A., Asiain, X., & Gorostiaga, E. M. (2006). Differential effects of strength training leading to failure versus not to failure on hormonal responses, strength, and muscle power gains. *Journal of Applied Physiology*, *100*, 1647-1656.

Jahreis, G., Kauf, E., Frohner, G., Schmidt, H. E. (1991). Influence of intensive exercise on insulin-like growth factor I, thyroid and steroid hormones in females gymnasts. *Growth Regul*, 95-99.

Kraemer, W. J. and Ratamess, N. A. (2005). Hormonal responses and adaptations to resistance exercise and training. *Sports Medecine*, 35, 339-361.

Lapachet, R. A., Miller, B. W. C. and Arnall, D. A. (1996). Body fat and exercise endurance in trained rats adapted to a high-fat diet and/or a high-carbohydrate diet *Journal of Applied Physiology,* 80, 1173-1179.

Levin, B. E., & Dunn-Meynell, A. A. (2004). Chronic exercise lowers the defended body weight gain and adiposity in diet-induced obese rats. *American Journal of Physiology, Regulatory, Integrative and Comparative Physiology*, *286*, R771-R778.

Liu, S., Baracos, V. E., Quinney, H. A., Clandinin, M. T. (1996). Dietary fat modifies exercise-dependent glucose transport in skeletal muscle. *J Appl Physiol.* 80, 1219-1224.

Mathey, J., Cavalié, H., Davicco, M. J., Coxam, V., Barlet, J. P., & Lac, G. (2000). Leptin and exercise. *Pflugers Archive*, *440*, R267.

Melanson, E. L., Gozansky, W. S., Barry, D. W., Maclean, P. S., Grunwald, G. K., & Hill, J. O. (2009). When energy balance is maintained, exercise does not induce negative fat balance in lean sedentary, obese sedentary, or lean endurance-trained individuals. *J Appl Physiol*, *107,* 1847-1856.

Périard, D., Folly, A., Meyer, M. A., Gautier, E., Krieg, M. A., & Hayoz, D. (2010). Aortic calcification and the risk of osteoporotic fractures. *Rev Med Suisse*, 7; 6 (271), 2200-2203.

Proulx, K., Vahl, T. P., Drazen, D. L., Woods, S. C., & Seeley, R. J. (2005). The effect of adrenalectomy on ghrelin secretion and orexgenic action. *Journal of Neuroendocrinology*, 17, 445-451.

Sacks, F. M., Bray, G. A., Carey, V. J., Smith, S. R., Ryan, D. H., Anton, S. D., et al. (2009). Comparison of weight-loss diets with different compositions on fat, protein, and carbohydrates. *N Engl J Med,* 360, 859-873.

Shai, I., Schwarzfuchs, D., Henkin, Y., Shahar, D.R., Witkow, S., Greenberg, I., et al. (2008). Weight loss with a low-carbohydrate, Mediterranean, or low-fat diet. *N Engl J Med*, *41*, 359-229.

Yaw, Y. H., Kandiah, M., Shariff, Z. M., Mun, C. Y., Hashim, Z., Yusof, R. M., Othman, Z., Saibul, N., & Weay, Y. H. (2010). Pattern of weight changes in women with breast cancer. *Asian Pac J Cancer Prev*, *11(6)*, 1535-1540.

INDEX

C

D

E

F

G

Q

R

S

T

U

V

W

Y